Quality and Risk Management in the IVF Laboratory

Second Edition

Quality and Risk Management in the IVF Laboratory

Second Edition

Sharon T. Mortimer, PhD
Director, Oozoa Biomedical Inc.
West Vancouver, BC, Canada

David Mortimer, PhD
President, Oozoa Biomedical Inc.
West Vancouver, BC, Canada

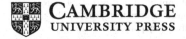

CAMBRIDGE
UNIVERSITY PRESS

CAMBRIDGE
UNIVERSITY PRESS

University Printing House, Cambridge CB2 8BS, United Kingdom

One Liberty Plaza, 20th Floor, New York, NY 10006, USA

477 Williamstown Road, Port Melbourne, VIC 3207, Australia

314-321, 3rd Floor, Plot 3, Splendor Forum, Jasola District Centre, New Delhi - 110025, India

79 Anson Road, #06-04/06, Singapore 079906

Cambridge University Press is part of the University of Cambridge.

It furthers the University's mission by disseminating knowledge in the pursuit of education, learning and research at the highest international levels of excellence.

www.cambridge.org
Information on this title: www.cambridge.org/9781107421288

First published 2005
Second edition 2015

A catalogue record for this publication is available from the British Library

Library of Congress Cataloging in Publication data
Mortimer, David, 1953– , author.
Quality and risk management in the IVF laboratory / Sharon T. Mortimer, David Mortimer. – Second edition.
    p. ; cm.
Authors' names reversed on the first edition.
ISBN 978-1-107-42128-8 (Paperback)
I. Mortimer, Sharon T. (Sharon Tracey), 1961– , author. II. Title.
[DNLM: 1. Fertilization in Vitro–standards. 2. Clinical Laboratory Techniques–standards. 3. Quality Control. 4. Risk Management–methods. WQ 208]
RG135
362.198′01780599–dc23 2014035094

ISBN 978-1-107-42128-8 Paperback

Contents

Introduction

In the introduction to the first edition of this book we commented that it seemed that we were hearing news reports of disasters in IVF clinics almost weekly, and that public concern over these reports had resulted in governments introducing regulation of IVF labs around the world. We also noted that within our profession there was growing recognition of the need for accreditation of IVF labs to minimize the potential for such errors to occur. In the intervening decade the prevalence of regulation has continued to increase, the acceptance of accreditation has become more widespread – and, gratifyingly, it seems that "IVF disasters" might have become less frequent. National and international professional societies have committees, working groups, special interest groups, and even task forces working in the area of quality management, risk management and safety in assisted reproductive technology (ART), and an increasing number of clinics now employ quality managers.

Quality systems, which have an inherent role in all modern accreditation schemes, are essentially based on the principles of ISO 9000 and related standards. Yet quality management beyond basic assay quality control is still often poorly understood by biomedical scientists, especially outside of clinical chemistry and pathology laboratories. In particular, even though risk analysis and minimization are being demanded of IVF labs, many IVF scientists have only limited understanding of how to go about these tasks. Ten years ago we suggested that this was because the majority of scientists working in clinical IVF labs had come from academic/research backgrounds and, as a consequence, had limited experience of the practicalities of laboratory management. However, it is still very obvious that too many IVF scientists receive little or no formal training in quality management – or even in the basics of laboratory management.

IVF continues its rapid evolution over the last four decades or so: from its beginnings as a highly experimental procedure in the late 1970s, culminating in the birth of Louise Brown on July 25, 1978 (Edwards and Steptoe, 1980) to a rapidly expanding field of research and a clinical practice that swept the world in the 1980s and was consolidated as a routine clinical service in the 1990s. From the mid-1980s we also saw the rapid growth in commercial IVF clinics, to the extent that IVF is often now described as an "industry" and IVF treatment (even ICSI) is increasingly seen by many as a commodity product, especially in the developed world. Over the last 15 years we have seen, at least in countries where the provision of ART services is more advanced, the "corporatization" of IVF clinics, with banks and other financial institutions now owning networks of clinics. Sadly the operation of such clinics now seems prone to being directed by finance professionals whose understanding and "feel" for the provision of quality ART care has been criticized in the mass media as being driven primarily by the motive of profit.

Nonetheless, even in the face of escalating global expansion and commercialization, quality management and risk management continue to increase in importance to those responsible for running IVF clinics, and consequently their understanding and practise by the scientists working in them becomes ever more important.

But quality management and risk management cannot be applied in isolation; they must be integrated within the holistic framework of total quality management, itself essentially synonymous with the goal of "best practice." In this way quality and risk management will not be seen as just additional annoying, expensive regulatory requirements that "don't help the patients get pregnant." The provision of effective and safe IVF treatment depends on achieving improved standards of technical services and medical care. Healthcare is slowly learning the lessons that transformed the manufacturing industries since World War II, and have done the same for service industries more recently. Within this context, calls for IVF centers to operate according to international standards such as ISO 9001 (Alper *et al.*, 2002; Alper, 2013) reflect modern awareness of our professional – and commercial – environment, and should be embraced by all centers that truly care for their patients and employees.

The structure and organization of IVF centers varies widely between small, "sole practitioner"-size clinics and large, corporate IVF organizations that typically operate multiple sites. Figure 1.1 shows a generic concept for viewing the organization of an IVF center by disciplines that is applicable to all clinics, regardless of size. The internal management of an IVF center is illustrated in Figure 1.2, establishing the appropriate levels of control necessary to operate a multidisciplinary organization that expresses mutual respect for all professions involved. IVF labs vary in size between a single scientist (we abhor the word "tech" or "technician" since we believe ardently that anyone performing IVF lab procedures *must* function as an autonomous professional scientist, but more of that later) and a large team that is often sub-divided by functions and responsibilities. These extremes are illustrated in the organization charts shown in Figures 1.3 and 1.4. A full understanding of organizational structure, the hierarchies of authority and responsibility, and lines of communication are essential pre-requisites for anyone embarking upon implementing programs of quality management and risk management.

Fortunately, each center does not need to re-invent the disciplines of quality management and risk management. Not only have numerous IVF centers around the world already achieved ISO 9001 certification, but the basic processes of managing quality improvement and risk management in IVF are not fundamentally different to other areas of business. There are many resources available to centers embarking upon this journey, ranging from "self-help" and reference books at all levels (we still refer to Dale and McQuater, 1998; Heller and Hindle, 2003; Hobbs, 2009), to practical advice from friendly centers, based upon their own experiences, to expert advice and assistance from commercially orientated centers, management companies, or individual consultants.

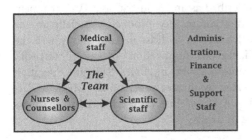

Figure 1.1 Diagrammatic representation of the organization of an IVF center showing the "core team" that must have effective administration, finance, and support teams working alongside it.

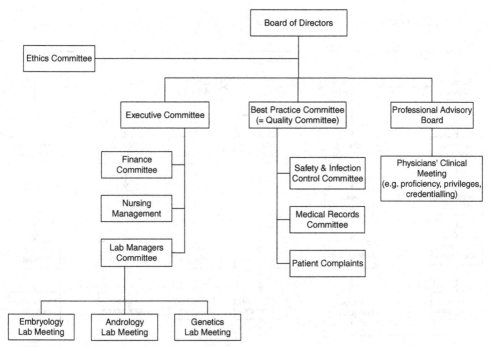

Figure 1.2 Organization chart showing the committee structure that might be required to run a large IVF center according to the principles of total quality management – or a generic accreditation scheme.

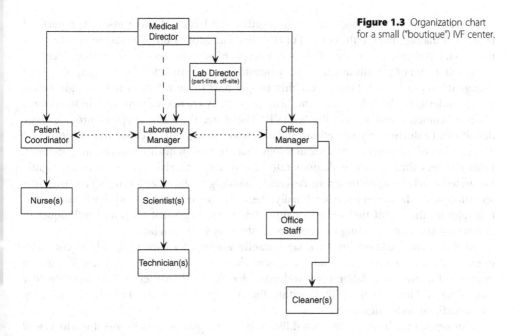

Figure 1.3 Organization chart for a small ("boutique") IVF center.

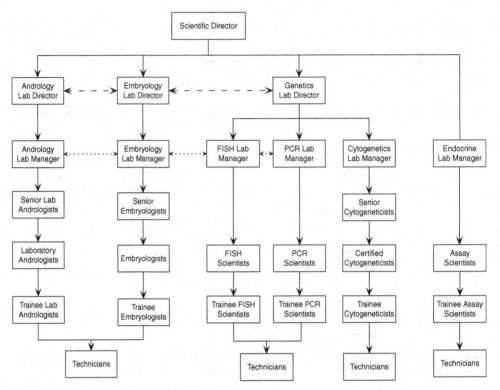

Figure 1.4 Organization chart for the laboratory operations of a large IVF center.

We have written this book to bring together the basics of these essential aspects of laboratory management in the context of IVF labs. The book is aimed at scientists who know their own technical field, but to whom the concepts of process and systems management are less familiar – if not actually alien. We see education as the foundation for bringing about any change or improvement. Simply teaching people how to do a task is not enough: unless people understand the "whys" (and the "why-nots") they are not truly competent to perform a job as complex and responsible as IVF. Therefore, the early chapters provide basic definitions (unfortunately sometimes didactic and boring, but essential nonetheless) and explanations of the concepts and terminology that are used in quality and risk management. Later chapters then go on to demonstrate how quality and risk management are tightly integrated in achieving optimum success rates, avoiding mistakes, and running an efficient – and successful – laboratory service. Finally, there are chapters that provide basic advice and examples on the use of the various quality and risk management tools and techniques in developing and implementing management systems in your own lab.

In this second edition we have significantly expanded Chapter 12, which considers human resource management, added a new chapter (13) that describes an illustrative example of a "well-run" laboratory, and expanded the final chapter (14) to now consider Total Quality Management (TQM) within the context of the entire IVF clinic, including cost-benefit considerations.

Throughout the book we have used illustrative examples from the general world as well as ones specific to the IVF lab. The latter often represent examples of what happens when things do go wrong: issues such as mis-matched sperm and eggs, transferring the wrong embryos, losing samples from the cryobank, letting cryobank tanks go dry and so on – painful as they might be for any of us to think about. Of course, there are examples of where things went right for us or our colleagues as well.

What happens when an IVF lab is "out of control"? The effects can be very varied, and not all aspects will appear at the same time (or ever), but some, many, or all of the following features will be revealed.

- Unpredictable and inexplicable variations in outcomes (and indicators, if they're being followed), with a likely general downward trend in results. In extreme cases things might deteriorate to such a state that the best description is that "the wheels have fallen off."
- That generalized perception that the feeling of "comfort" that you had when things were running smoothly fades, and ultimately a sense of panic (controlled or not) might eventuate.
- Everyone starts to get "defensive" and this can deteriorate into fault-finding, "finger-pointing," and blame. If this is not checked then a general culture of fear, blame, and retribution can develop, and the lab (and, by then, probably the whole clinic) can become a "toxic workplace."

If you recognize any of these symptoms in your lab or clinic then you should definitely read on!

When we were asked to sum up what the first edition of this book would be about, and what its focus would be, we synthesized our concepts and ideas, our beliefs and attitudes, as well as summarizing our then combined 60 years of practical experience in the field into the simple statement of "taking a holistic approach to prophylactic management" – achieving prevention rather than cure. For the revised and expanded second edition we have retained this basic philosophy, which has only been strengthened over the past decade.

Regulation, licensing, and accreditation

What's the difference?

Regulation, licensing, and accreditation are often confused with each other, or seen as alternative viewpoints on how IVF labs are governed. In fact, they are different concepts and all three must work together within an integrated system of governance. Let's start with some definitions.

Regulations: These are legal requirements[1] to which an organization or individual must conform in order to operate. Compliance is often verified by inspection (examination for individuals) and confirmed by the issuance of a license. Regulations are typically highly prescriptive as to what an organization or individual must/must not do in order to be compliant.

Accreditation: This is a collegial process based on self- and peer-assessment whereby an authoritative body (usually a non-government organization) gives formal recognition that an organization is in voluntary compliance with one or more Standards set by the authoritative body. Unlike licensing, accreditation is based upon process rather than procedure, and the principles of quality improvement rather than strict obedience of regulations, so that it is not prescriptive in relation to technical procedures or rules. The end result of an accreditation process (being "accredited") is often termed certification or registration by the authoritative body.

Licensing: This is the process whereby an organization (or individual) is identified as being compliant with required regulations. Usually, licensing is a legal requirement under government regulations in order for an organization to be allowed to operate (*c.f.* certification). For individuals, licensing is conferred to denote their competence to perform a given activity (e.g. driving a motor vehicle) in compliance with regulations.

Some other terms that are heard or seen in discussions of regulation, licensing, and accreditation that, unless used properly and not synonymously, include "certification" and "credentialling" (*c.f.* "licensing"), "standards" as compared to "regulations," and "inspection" versus "survey." Again, some more definitions:

---

[1] *A requirement is a need or expectation that can be either stated explicitly, customarily implied, or obligatory (i.e. a regulation).*

Certification: This is the process whereby an organization (or individual) is identified as meeting one or more selected standards. The term is essentially synonymous with "registration" in the ISO system. A certification report will typically highlight any areas of non-conformance and require changes that "must" be made in order to achieve certification, as well as recommendations or suggestions of changes that the organization "should" or "could" make to improve its operations (*c.f.* licensing).

Several national societies have developed certification schemes for clinical embryologists, e.g. the UK Association of Clinical Embryologists, Australia's Scientists in Reproductive Technology, the College of Reproductive Biology (a special interest group within the American Association of Bioanalysts) in the USA, and the ART Lab Special Interest Group of the Canadian Fertility and Andrology Society. These schemes award certificates to personnel based on their competence, evaluated against a set of required competencies developed by their peers, and hence can also been seen as a credentialling process (see below).

Going beyond this, in the Netherlands, only KLEM-certified embryologists can work in a legislated Dutch IVF lab (KLEM = Vereniging voor Klinische Embryologie, the Dutch Society for Clinical Embryology), and some countries have also implemented regulatory schemes that include the certification of clinical embryologists, e.g. the New Zealand Health Practitioners Competence Assurance Act of 2003. In the UK, as of October 2013, the well-developed ACE Certificate scheme was superseded by a Government (NHS) postgraduate entry-only Scientist Training Program, leading to registration with the Health and Care Professions Council.

Credentialling: This is a process for assigning specific responsibilities (or "scope of practice") to individual professionals based on their training, qualifications, experience and current practice (actual expertise) within an organizational framework. It is an employer's responsibility, with a professional development focus, that commences upon appointment and continues throughout each individual's employment. Credentialling is based on verifying that an individual meets an expected set of competencies that have been defined by their peers and are designed to ensure quality of practice and management of risk; in medicine, credentialling is sometimes referred to as "clinical governance."

Inspection: This is a process carried out by one or more authorized inspectors, to determine whether an organization or facility conforms to a defined set of regulations. Inspection is typically a requirement for licensing under regulations.

Standards: These are published documents that contain technical specifications or criteria to be used consistently as rules, guidelines, or definitions of characteristics to ensure that materials, products, processes, and services are fit for their purpose. Unlike a regulation, a Standard is a "living document" that describes a voluntary agreement between all stakeholders relevant to the product or service, and encompasses everything that can have a profound influence on the product or service, especially its safety, reliability, and efficiency. Compliance with Standards is ascertained through a process of assessment or accreditation, rather than inspection. These Standards are not synonymous with "minimum standards," which, while they define the minimum technical requirements for a process to be performed or undertaken, do not usually consider anything beyond basic quality control (i.e. do not consider quality improvement or the quality cycle, see Chapter 3).

Survey: This is the preferred term for the visit to a facility or organization that is being assessed for accreditation. A survey typically follows a self-assessment process by the organization and is performed by a (typically) multidisciplinary survey team that evaluates the organization's progress towards the goals described in the Standards. (See "A generic accreditation process," below).

Regulation and licensing of IVF

Regulation and licensing are systems that are imposed on an organization, such as a clinical laboratory or an IVF center. These systems, which are not optional, are usually created and enforced via legislation and consequently vary widely between countries, and even between states in countries such as Australia and the USA. Licensing bodies (e.g. the Human Fertilisation and Embryology Authority, the HFEA, in the UK) typically issue a licence after an inspection process to confirm that an organization is, indeed, operating in accordance with the law. While this process does create some sort of minimum standards to which the facility or organization will operate, there is often no consideration of performance standards or quality within the terms of the licensing process.

The European Union Tissues and Cells Directive (EUTCD) 2004/23/EC seeks to set "standards of quality and safety for the donation, procurement, testing, processing, preservation, storage and distribution of human tissues and cells," with practical matters relating to donation procurement and testing being covered in a 1st Technical Directive (2006/17/EC), and operational technical requirements being covered in a 2nd Technical Directive (2006/86/EC). Together these three directives provide a framework for the operation of tissue banks across the EU, including IVF labs. Member states have since incorporated these directives into their national legal laws, and have each conferred regulatory authority on a national agency for their implementation and operation, e.g. the UK HFEA, the Irish Medicines Board, and the French Agence de Biomédecine.

Regulation and licensing are therefore not particularly relevant to the focus of this book, and will be left for other authors to explore. Instead, our focus will be on the setting of – and complying with – Standards that go beyond meeting minimum standards, an approach that can be described simplistically as seeking to achieve best practice. The formalization of such an approach is usually referred to as certification or accreditation. As defined above, "certification" is typically used when referring to standards such as ISO Standards (see below), while "accreditation" is a more broad-based approach founded upon a perpetual process of quality improvement.

As a final word, we must all be aware of other regulations that we are obliged to follow in any workplace:

- Regulations that affect the employer/employee relationship, such as those that create statutory requirements pertaining to maximum work hours, statutory holidays, annual leave, etc. Labor relations in general is an area that no employer can ignore – if for no other reason than a disgruntled employee will be sure to remind him/her of them!
- The handling and use of hazardous materials such as flammable solvents, strong acids and alkalis, liquid nitrogen, radioactive materials, etc. All materials used in the IVF lab must be stored, handled, and used correctly for the safety of everyone – and the facility. For example, in Canada the Workplace Hazardous Materials Information System (WHMIS) is designed to reduce the risk from hazardous products in the workplace at all levels (i.e. suppliers, workers, and employers) through proper training and the requirement that a Material Safety Data Sheet (MSDS) for each product must be available to anyone who comes into contact with it.
- General occupational health and safety.
- Fire regulations.
- Building codes.

Add to this the complexities of the EUTCD, for example, and there is a veritable minefield of regulation that affects almost everything we do, from designing a lab to how high a fire extinguisher can be placed above the floor! Just because someone works in a (small) private IVF lab and, in their opinion, "something-or-other doesn't matter here," does not give them any right to break such regulations. Ignore them at your peril!

Accreditation

As defined already, accreditation is a voluntary, collegial process based on self- and peer-assessment whereby an authoritative body (usually a non-government organization) gives formal recognition that an organization is complying to an acceptable degree with one or more Standards set by the non-government body. Accreditation is based on process rather than procedure, and the principles of quality improvement rather than strict obedience of regulations. An accreditation scheme is not prescriptive in relation to any technical procedures or rules.

Accreditation Standards are most definitely not "minimum standards." Minimum standards only define the essential technical requirements for a process to be performed or undertaken, including the basic quality control procedures necessary to ensure that it has been done correctly; they do not usually consider quality improvement or the quality cycle (see Chapter 3).

Accreditation Standards contain the technical specifications or criteria that must be applied consistently – whether as rules, guidelines, or definitions of characteristics – to ensure that materials, products, processes, and services are fit for their purpose. Moreover, an accreditation Standard describes a voluntary agreement between all parties involved in the product or service, and it encompasses every component or factor that can influence the product or service, especially its safety, reliability, and efficiency. Because our understanding of the processes by which we create a product or provide a service grow with experience, it is vital that an accreditation Standard be a "living document." Processes are dynamic and therefore Standards cannot be embodied within legislation that will probably take years to modify or reform.

Determining whether an organization is complying with an agreed set of accreditation Standards involves a process of assessment and evaluation that typically includes a self-assessment exercise in advance of a *survey* (not an "inspection" or "assessment" site visit) by a multidisciplinary team of surveyors who have received specialized training in reviewing an organization's systems and processes – both as generalized concepts and with specialist, industry-specific knowledge and experience. The organization seeking accreditation is supplied with a set of descriptive Standards against which it can evaluate itself and then submit a preliminary self-assessment. After review of this document, a survey team is sent out to review the organization and its operations and assess their compliance with the Standards and their progress towards achieving their goals.

The following are examples of accreditation schemes:

Australia: The Reproductive Technology Accreditation Committee or "RTAC," which operates under the aegis of the Fertility Society of Australia. RTAC accreditation (now achieved via audit by an independent certifying body under the Joint Accreditation Scheme of Australia and New Zealand [JAS-ANZ]) is required for all IVF units in Australia in order for their patients to receive Medicare rebates for IVF treatment and to access gonadotrophins under the Government's Pharmaceutical Benefits Scheme. IVF centers in New Zealand also participate in the RTAC accreditation scheme.

Australia: The National Association of Testing Authorities or "NATA" accredits all testing facilities including medical laboratories, which are accredited according to ISO 15189. Although IVF units are not required to have NATA accreditation, several have sought this independent accreditation. However, any laboratory performing diagnostic testing (e.g. andrology or endocrine) must be NATA accredited.

Australia: Australian Council on Healthcare Standards or "ACHS" is a non-government organization that accredits hospitals and healthcare organizations.

Canada: Accreditation Canada (previously the Canadian Council on Health Services Accreditation or "CCHSA") is a non-government organization that accredits hospitals and healthcare organizations. An accreditation scheme for IVF clinics was developed jointly with the Canadian Fertility and Andrology Society (CFAS) in the early 2000s within what was then the CCHSA's "AIM" program (Achieving Improved Measurement), and then revised to come under Accreditation Canada's "Qmentum" program in 2010.

UK: Clinical Pathology Accreditation (UK) Ltd or "CPA" is a non-government organization that accredits medical laboratories. It also operates several external quality assurance (EQA) schemes.

With the development of the 7th edition of its code of practice, published in 2007, the HFEA took the unusual step of integrating accreditation principles with its licensing requirements, combining the HFE Act 1990 and the EUTCD, along with embracing the principles of ISO 9001 and ISO 15189.

USA: The College of American Pathologists or "CAP" operates a voluntary Reproductive Laboratory Accreditation Program (RLAP) that was developed in conjunction with the American Society for Reproductive Medicine (ASRM). However, this program only applies to laboratories performing andrology tests regulated by CLIA'88; IVF centers are not accredited by the CAP RLAP.

USA: The Joint Commission on Accreditation of Healthcare Organizations or "JCAHO" is an independent, not-for-profit organization that considers itself to be the nation's predominant standards-setting and accrediting body in healthcare. JCAHO accredits all types of laboratories and healthcare organizations, including IVF labs.

Beyond these national accreditation schemes there is international accreditation by the International Organization for Standardization, commonly known as "ISO," whose Standards are being increasingly seen as the "gold standard" for IVF clinics.

ISO standards

The International Organization for Standardization (www.iso.ch) or "ISO" is based in Geneva and develops standards according to the essential principles of:

consensus – the views of all interested parties are taken into account: manufacturers, vendors and users, consumer groups, testing laboratories, governments, engineering professions, and research organizations;

industry-wide – they are global solutions intended to satisfy industries and customers worldwide; and

voluntary – international standardization is market-driven and therefore based on the voluntary involvement of all interests in the marketplace.

The following ISO standards are relevant to IVF centers and their laboratories.

The ISO 9000 family of standards

The first edition of the ISO 9000 series of standards for quality management and quality assurance was released in 1987, at which time they were known in the various member countries by their own designation (e.g. BS 5750 in the UK). The second edition was introduced in 1994 when most countries made their numbering compatible with the ISO system:

1. ISO 9001:1994 *Quality Systems – Model for Quality Assurance in Design, Development, Production, Installation and Servicing.* This standard was essentially directed towards manufacturers.

2. ISO 9002:1994 *Quality Systems – Model for Quality Assurance in Production, Installation and Servicing.* This standard was very similar to ISO 9001:1994 but had no requirements for design control, being aimed essentially at service organizations.

3. ISO 9003–1994 *Quality Systems – Model for Quality Assurance in Final Inspection and Test.* This standard was intended for quality testing organizations.

For the third (2000) edition, ISO 9002 and ISO 9003 were withdrawn, leaving just one standard for certification: ISO 9001:2000. This single quality management system requirement standard replaced the three quality assurance requirement standards ISO 9001:1994, ISO 9002:1994, and ISO 9003:1994. ISO 9001:2000 was developed to assist organizations of all types and sizes to implement and operate an effective quality management system (QMS) based on a more process-based approach, including an expectation of processes for ensuring continuous improvement.

Therefore, ISO 9001:2000 specifies requirements for a user-defined QMS that will allow an organization to demonstrate its ability to provide products that meet customer requirements and applicable regulatory requirements, and aims to enhance customer satisfaction. Organizations can exclude certain requirements of the standard if some of its clauses are not relevant to their quality systems.

The ISO 9000 family now comprises four core standards that form a coherent set of QMS standards facilitating mutual understanding in national and international trade (see http://www.iso.org/iso/iso_9000):

1. ISO 9000:2005 *Quality Management Systems – Fundamentals and Vocabulary*, covering the basic concepts and language.
2. ISO 9001:2008 *Quality Management Systems – Requirement*, which sets out the requirements of a quality management system. ISO 9001 *Quality Management Systems* is currently under review, with an updated version expected by the end of 2015.
3. ISO 9004:2009 *Managing for the Sustained Success of an Organization – A Quality Management Approach*. This document focuses on how to make a quality management system more efficient and effective. It provides guidelines for both effectiveness and efficiency based upon the fundamental aim of improving the performance of an organization and the satisfaction of customers and other interested parties.
4. ISO 19011:2011 *Guidelines for Auditing Management Systems*, providing guidance on internal and external audits of quality management systems.

ISO standards for laboratories

For laboratories there are other, specific ISO standards that affect them. Until the early 2000s this was the ISO standard applicable to all laboratories (ISO/IEC 17025:2000 *General Requirements for the Competence of Testing and Calibration Laboratories*; now ISO 17025:2005), but for medical laboratories it was superseded by ISO 15189:2003 *Medical Laboratories – Particular Requirements for Quality and Competence*, now ISO 15189:2012. This new standard specifically considers the provision of laboratory-based medical services and is, therefore, the relevant ISO standard for andrology and IVF labs.

Therefore, while IVF centers might choose to be accredited according to ISO 9001:2008, their laboratory activities must (also) comply with ISO 15189:2012.

A generic accreditation process

Accreditation can be viewed as a structured means of achieving positive organizational change, rather than change being enforced through an adversarial process. Usually, the accrediting authority is a non-governmental organization or not-for-profit company that has developed, in consultation with the professional bodies and other stakeholders involved in the particular field, a set of Standards that represent the consensus opinion as to operational standards and performance in the field. Effective accreditation schemes around the world share the same three basic characteristics (see Figure 2.1):

1. Self-study/evaluation/assessment;
2. External assessment via a survey by peers; and
3. Recommendations.

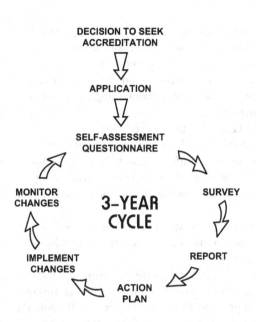

Figure 2.1 A generic accreditation process.

Self-assessment

An initial self-assessment by the organization is at the heart of accreditation. The organization undertakes a comprehensive examination of all aspects of its mission, programs and services, a process that necessarily involves individuals from every area and level of the organization, as well as the organization's customers (patients and referrers) and, ideally, the public. Input from all these "stakeholders" is used to create a detailed self-assessment report documenting the organization's current status quo.

Sometimes, during preparation for the self-assessment phase, on-site focus group consultations might be held that allow surveyors (not necessarily the ones who will undertake the actual formal survey of the organization) to meet with staff, patients, and the organization's community stakeholders. The goal of these meetings is to help increase communication and collaboration throughout the organization, and thereby improve the validity of the self-assessment exercise's findings. The self-assessment process has the following goals:

- to determine compliance with established accreditation criteria or "Standards";
- to assess the organization's alignment with its own stated philosophies and goals, as well as those that might be imposed by any regulatory authority, in terms of patient care and the delivery of service;
- to evaluate outcomes and effectiveness; and
- to identify, and prioritize, areas for improvement.

A major benefit that flows from the self-assessment process is the "buy-in" to the process from everyone involved ("Building a Process Map" in Chapter 5).

Typical accreditation Standards cover the following operational areas of the organization, across which the concepts of "education for life" and "achieving best results" are overarching philosophical principles.

- **Governance:** Including management structure and responsibility, leadership issues, partnerships with and accountability towards other stakeholders, ethical issues, risk management, and perhaps even the organization's financial soundness.
- **Human resources:** Identifying and addressing needs, attracting and keeping the right people (including career development issues), creating and maintaining good working relationships, as well as a healthy work environment.
- **Information management:** Collecting and keeping data, data security, and confidentiality, and the use of data in benchmarking, decision-making, and research.
- **Information technology:** The application and use of information technology, not only in relation to information management, but also operational efficiency, continuing education and career development for managers and staff, and educational material for patients.
- **Environmental:** Providing a suitable environment for staff and patients, as well as for the procedures and services being performed, minimizing the occurrence of adverse events, and respect for the environment in general.
- **Clinical services:** The provision of patient care, including diagnostic work-up, the delivery of therapeutic services and subsequent follow-up (often termed the "continuum of care"); competent and responsive clinical practices that meet the needs of the patients in particular and the community (society) in general, including the consent process and respecting patients' rights; continuing education for medical and related staff (nurse coordinators, counsellors, etc.) and also patients.
- **Laboratory services:** General compliance with good laboratory practice ("GLP"), adequate and appropriately designed space, having, operating, and maintaining adequate and suitable equipment, using appropriate and suitable reagents and other products, as well as the general technical procedures involved in the handling, culturing, and cryopreservation of gametes and embryos.

External assessment

After the self-assessment exercise, a site visit by a team of surveyors from outside the organization seeking accreditation is scheduled to assess the strengths and weaknesses of the organization. The survey team comprises a group of objective professionals who have received special training in performing such surveys. During the survey they will view the premises, meet with management, conduct interviews with members of staff and (willing) patients, and examine data to determine whether the organization is in compliance with the accrediting authority's established criteria or Standards. The survey team would typically conduct an "exit interview" to present its findings and might offer some preliminary advice from what will be included in its written report.

A draft report is then submitted by the survey team to the accrediting authority's board or management for review and approval. The accrediting authority then passes the approved official report and recommendations on to the organization's management.

Assessment results and recommendations

The findings from the survey, including their analysis in relation to the self-assessment document, are summarized in a written report whose purpose is to focus on the organization's strengths and weaknesses. Recommendations are made to help the organization develop plans, not only to improve areas where they are weak, but also to maintain and expand areas where they are strong. Recommendations in a survey report follow a standardized code of expression that allows the organization seeking accreditation to interpret them:

Must or *shall*	denote recommendations that are considered necessary for the organization to become compliant with a particular Standard, or alleviate a recognized problem.
Should	denotes recommendations which, in the light of the surveyors' experience, will improve the organization's rating according to a particular Standard, or are likely to provide significant benefit to the organization's operational standards or performance (although they might be subject to prioritization by the organization's management or its governing body).
Could	identifies suggestions for changes that might, in light of the surveyors' experience and/or that of other similar organizations, improve the organization's operational standards or performance, and would be expected to generate an improvement in the organization's rating according to a particular Standard.

The recommendations are then used to create an action plan (sometimes divided into phases so as not to be overwhelming), which is how change will be effected.

Afterwards

Accreditation is not a cyclical process. While the surveys might well run on a three-year cycle, quality does not. Quality must be ongoing; through continuous quality improvement, it is a perpetual process built upon the quality cycle (see Chapter 3). Certainly, everyone deserves a break after completing all the exhausting preparations for a survey visit and surviving the survey visit itself (especially the first time around!) – but just for a few hours or a day (just enough time for a party, perhaps). But there should never be any need for anyone to have to "get back" into the quality management program – because by then the whole thing should be tightly integrated into the daily functioning of every part of the clinic (*not* just the lab).

Quality must be integral, it can't be an add-on, and any organization that relaxes its commitment to quality and considers that it doesn't have to worry about "accreditation stuff" until the time comes around to prepare their next self-assessment, has simply failed to see the point of accreditation, and will certainly not reap the full benefit of everyone's hard work.

The need to use your own processes

When developing a quality management system, it is vital that you develop and use your own processes rather than try to follow somebody else's rules. Every IVF lab or IVF center is different. There will be local permutations or variations in practice that will preclude you blindly following a system or process that you have "borrowed" from another clinic. Certainly you can base your methods and systems on those from another IVF lab, but unless you intend to copy that entire center in the most minute detail, you will always have to adapt them. This subject is discussed in more detail in Chapters 5 and 6.

Quality and quality management

What is quality?

Traditionally, quality was seen as an expression of the superiority of a product, meaning that it might work better, or last longer, or just look nicer. Usually, higher-grade materials were used and more care was put into its manufacture and finish, with the result that a quality product cost more money, but this was worth it if one took into account its attributes – and, of course, if one could afford the extra cost. But quality is not the same as luxury, which represents opulence, i.e. products that are better than they need to be to serve their primary purpose, and is typically more expensive. After all, even if you are a successful sales rep with a large territory you don't *need* a Rolls Royce for driving around the countryside – but you *do* need a car that doesn't break down, is preferably not too fuel hungry, and is comfortable (because you'll spend several hours each day sitting in it).

From a basic product-manufacturing perspective, quality can be defined as *conformance to specifications* – specifications that are set by the manufacturer, based on the manufacturer's experience of what the customer wanted. This can, of course, be discovered by carrying out customer surveys or by looking at sales figures. But in service industries the concept of quality is rather more difficult to define. Again, businesses have tried to define their best quality efforts (i.e. the quality of their services) according to certain specifications, usually ones that management have defined and then refined – hopefully as a result of seeking the opinions and approval of their customers.

A major advance in understanding the concept of quality comes when it is defined as *fitness for use* – with the focus being orientated completely towards the customers' perceptions and opinions. Sometimes this change in perspective is described as a switch from being a "product-out" company to a "market-in" company. Another description of this approach is *conformance to customer requirements*, as opposed to the earlier *conformance to [manufacturer] specifications*.

Quality management

Quality management is the integration of quality activities, which include quality control, quality assurance, and quality improvement, into a management philosophy. Historically, quality management has its roots in the re-birth of the Japanese manufacturing industry after World War II, when Japan had a reputation for producing some of the worst manufactured goods in the world. However, by the 1960s Japanese products were often the highest quality ones in various market areas. This philosophy of total quality control was taught in Japan by W. Edwards Deming, PhD and Joseph M. Juran, BSEE, JD, and when it was embraced by Western companies and organizations in the 1980s and 1990s it became known as total quality management, or TQM. All these quality management systems share common roots, and an overview of the more commonly encountered systems has been provided later in this chapter. For many experts, TQM is simply *the scientific way of doing business* – so it is ideally suited to running an IVF lab.

Deming made a very important statement about quality and its modern application: *Good quality does not necessarily mean high quality. It means a predictable degree of uniformity and dependability with a quality suited to the market.* But in medicine we must expand our horizons and go beyond just applying concepts that relate to manufacturing industries.

In medicine, quality can also be defined as *duty of care* and has been equated to the achievement of *best practice.* For an IVF lab, these definitions can be combined with *conformance to customer requirements* to establish a framework that embraces the provision of quality services that not only meet the customers' needs, but also their expectations. From a holistic perspective, these services must also be effective, efficient, and safe, while protecting the rights and dignity of all parties involved – including the children who will result from successful treatment. It is also worth noting that "customers" include not only the patients, but also other referring doctors and healthcare providers (e.g. NHS Trusts in the UK, or HMOs in the United States).

Terminology

As in all specialized areas of expert knowledge, TQM has a wealth of terminology that must be used correctly to communicate one's ideas and intentions clearly with others, and also to avoid the confusion that arises from the incorrect use of terms. The most commonly used terms in TQM are defined below:

Quality assurance: "QA" is the entirety of systematic activities implemented within a quality system (i.e. including QC) that are necessary to provide adequate confidence that a product or service will satisfy its required quality characteristics.

Quality control: "QC" is the establishment of quality specifications for each quality characteristic, assessment of procedures used to determine conformance to these specifications, and taking any necessary corrective actions to bring them into conformance; for example, ensuring that an assay procedure has been performed correctly and that its result is within the (pre-defined) acceptable limits of uncertainty of measurement (see Chapter 6).

Quality cycle: This is a repeated cycle, often expressed graphically, of quality improvement in relation to a single product or service (a.k.a. "continuous quality improvement").

Quality improvement: "QI" is that part of a quality system focused on continually increasing effectiveness and efficiency. "Continuous quality improvement" is when QI is progressive and the organization actively seeks and pursues quality improvement opportunities.

Quality management: This describes the sum of all activities of the overall management function that determine the quality policy, objectives, and responsibilities, and implementation of them by means such as quality planning, quality control, quality assurance, and quality improvement within a defined quality system.

Quality management system: "QMS" describes the entire system developed by an organization involving the establishment of a quality policy and quality objectives and the processes to achieve those objectives.

Quality manager: This is the individual within an organization charged with achieving quality, and who is given the authority (and resources) to pursue it; the senior manager responsible for the organization's quality system.

Quality manual: This document describes an organization's quality management system.

Quality objective: This is something that is sought, or aimed for, in relation to creating or defining quality.

Quality planning: The part of quality management that is focused on setting quality objectives and specifying the necessary operational processes and related resources to fulfill quality objectives.

Quality policy: The overall intentions and directions of an organization, as specified by management, related to the fulfilment of quality requirements.

Quality system: The organizational structure, procedures, processes, and resources for implementing quality management.

Total quality management: The management approach of an organization, centered on quality and based on the participation of all its members, that aims at long-term success through customer satisfaction and creating benefits to all its members and to society.

An example of quality in action

Consider a company that manufactures TVs. The company receives many complaints from its customers that the TV sets they buy do not work when they get them home. The company realizes that 3 out of every 10 sets that it makes are apparently faulty – and is deeply concerned that very soon word of the customer complaints will spread and no-one will buy their product any more. So they install a man at the end of the production line whose job is to plug each TV set into a power outlet and check that it works before packing it into its carton: a quality control (QC) inspector. Very soon the complaints stop and customer satisfaction is at 100% – problem solved!

But, the company's financial controller soon realizes that 30% of their raw materials costs and 30% of their manufacturing costs are going entirely to waste, being tossed into a skip out behind the factory and sent to the garbage dump. Such waste represents a very large part of the company's profit margin – and it can't go on. So, the non-working TVs are taken apart and the reasons why they don't work are identified and tabulated. The most common cause is found, perhaps a problem with soldering on the main circuit board, and the problem rectified. Now the QC inspector only has to reject 3 sets out of every 20 – the proportion of "good" TVs is now 85% instead of 70% – a major saving in costs.

However, the financial controller is still not happy because profits are still not great and therefore insists that the next most common reason for sets not working also be remedied, which, in due course, it is. Now only 1 in 20 of the TV sets coming off the production line doesn't work: the waste is down to 5% and the proportion of "good" TVs is 95% – wonderful news! But the cost of employing the QC inspector is now greater than the cost of the wasted parts and labor and so the financial controller recommends that he be made redundant and the 5% wastage be written off.

Fortunately for the QC inspector, the owner of the company believes that 5% of his customers being angry is still too many – after all, they might tell their friends about their bad experience and then they'll buy their next TVs from another company. The owner decides to keep on the QC inspector until the manufacturing problems have been reduced to less than 1% – and so the engineers keep dealing with the less and less frequent manufacturing problems until they have reached the owner's target. Coincidentally, just at that time there happens to be a vacancy on the production line so the QC inspector gets a better job, making sure that all the components that are delivered to the assemblers are correct and that they never run out, which would slow down production.

End result: the company now has a much better quality product, more than 99% of their customers are satisfied with their new TV sets, the company is more profitable than ever, the owner is happy, the financial controller gets a bonus and the ex-QC inspector has a better, more secure job. And everyone is absolutely convinced that "quality pays."

Going beyond QC and QA: the quality cycle

In industry *quality control* focuses on inspection and checking, its purpose is to reduce waste, and it uses inspectors to check the work of others. In a laboratory, QC typically equates to making sure an assay was run properly: calibrators are used to ensure instruments are working properly, reference standards are used to verify that the results come out close to where they should. QC is about making sure each task is done correctly.

In all areas of endeavor, *quality assurance* focuses on procedures and systems. Quality is designed into a process, thereby increasing the likelihood that when the particular method is followed, the process will go exactly as planned, increasing consistency and overall performance. In other words, QA relates to the *way* in which work is done.

The *quality cycle* (see Figure 3.1) is a process whereby an issue or problem is recognized, a solution identified and put into effect, and the outcome checked to ensure that the issue or problem has been resolved. The cycle can be repeated if the issue is a complex one and there are several solutions to its component problems.

Figure 3.1 The quality cycle.

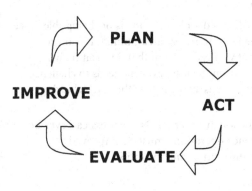

Continuous quality improvement: the ultimate goal

Quality describes the goal of satisfying requirements. But requirements change as customers' expectations rise, a perfectly normal situation that results from the essential spirit of competition that is inherent in the human psyche. To attract customers, a business has to offer more of something, or charge less. Charging less is an asymptotic process due to such realities as raw materials costs, labor costs, wholesale prices, etc., and once economies of scale have been realized there is no room to create further competitive edge. So, businesses must offer more for the same price – or at least a price that their customers perceive as having good value to them and being worth the price difference.

In IVF we have decidedly fixed costs in terms of consumables such as plasticware, culture media, oocyte retrieval needles, and embryo transfer catheters, and given the shortage of skilled embryologists there is essentially a "seller's market" for labor, so salaries must be competitive and hence are more likely to go up than be amenable to savings. So we must offer "more" to our patients, for example:

- more zygotes for a given number of oocytes;
- more embryos that are suitable for transfer or freezing in each treatment cycle;
- higher implantation potential for each fresh embryo transferred;
- higher oocyte/embryo cryosurvival; and
- higher implantation potential for each thawed/warmed embryo transferred.

In other words we must optimize our IVF/ICSI fertilization rates, our embryo culture systems, and our cryopreservation techniques. Then, within the context of the IVF center, we must make those services more easily available, provide them in a more pleasant environment and with more personalized attention. Finally, our more effective services must be provided in a more efficient manner: i.e. in the private sector we must maximize our profit margins, in the public sector we must control costs so more treatment can be provided within a given budget. This is what *total quality* is about: *continuously improving customer satisfaction levels and simultaneously improving margins.*

With "buy-in" from the team our goal becomes *the achievement of total quality through everyone's commitment and involvement* – a common definition for *total quality management.* But creating a work environment where continuous quality improvement can flourish depends on proper leadership.

Leadership of continuous quality improvement

There are three basic principles of leadership:

Challenge: This can be summarized as the need for long-term vision, being able to see the challenges that must be faced to realize an ambition. It is more important to recognize what we need to learn than just stating what needs to be done. Everyone, from the leader down, needs to challenge themselves every day, asking themselves whether they are achieving their goals.

Improvement: Embrace the adage "good enough never is." No process can ever be considered perfect, and hence operations must be improved continuously, striving for innovation and evolution.

Participation: It is vital that leaders go to the source to see the facts for themselves; having all the right facts is essential for making the right decisions, creating consensus, and making sure goals are attained at the best possible speed.

Effective leaders have and show respect for their people, and employ a management style that can be defined according to two simple principles:

Respect: Taking every stakeholder's problems seriously, and making every effort to build mutual trust. Taking responsibility for enabling other people to achieve their objectives.

Teamwork: Developing individuals through team problem-solving. Developing and engaging people through their contribution to team performance.

Leadership in general is considered in more detail in Chapter 12 "Human resources".

Total quality management

While there are many definitions of TQM, they all share the common perspective of it being a philosophy rather than a simple management procedure. It must be seen as a process of improvement beyond the status quo that then extends into an all-encompassing program of developing, and fostering, the desire for change and improvement throughout the entire organization. TQM is an all-encompassing quality system. It includes QC, QA, and QI within a perpetual reiterative process, but it is still based upon the foundations of inspection and audit (see Figure 3.2). TQM must be seen as a long-term goal, there are no short cuts or quick fixes in implementing TQM. There is no tool or technique that can be seen as a panacea for all the problems and woes of an organization, no turn-key systems that can be plugged into an organization's pre-existing management structure. Achieving a system of continuous improvement can take years, depending on the nature and size of the organization: time frames of 8 to 10 years have been suggested for big corporations, although from experience the more limited nature of even a big IVF center can allow success within two or three years.

TQM in IVF can be seen as encompassing the following areas of a center's operation, all of which impinge upon the laboratory:

- **Medical and scientific standards:** Obviously the latest and best techniques and protocols are required to enable the medical and laboratory staff to provide the highest-quality services to patients. This can be summed up as striving to achieve "best practice."
- **Responsibility:** Everyone involved in IVF must have a sense of responsibility for their actions. The fundamental principle of medicine, *primum non nocere* or "first do no harm" must always be uppermost in everyone's minds.
- **Duty of care:** There is a clear, and inescapable, duty of care towards not just the patients being treated, but also to the future children who will be created by successful treatment.
- **Ethics:** A great deal has been written and said about ethics in assisted reproduction technology, which ranges from simple artificial insemination on the one hand to reproductive cloning on the other. The vast majority of practitioners, both medical and scientific, have extremely high ethical standards, but it only takes the odd

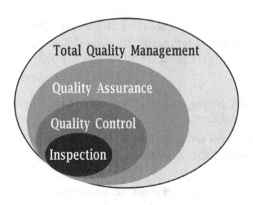

Figure 3.2 A diagrammatic overview of total quality management.

person who is determined to challenge society, or "push the envelope," to create headlines and bring everyone else under suspicion. Ethics must be seen as existing at several levels:

- *Personal ethics*, which can be moral or religious (although these can be considered more as "beliefs" that do not necessarily have any foundation in science);
- *Professional ethics*, often consisting of codes of conduct or recommendations for good practice produced by professional bodies; and
- *Society also has ethical perspectives*, and these are embodied in the requirement for ethics committees or institutional review boards – which can be seen as either a normal obligation stemming from our existence within a developed society or as a requirement imposed by regulatory bodies.

- **Customer expectations:** In IVF, as in any service industry, our customers – both the patients to whom we provide treatment and the other professionals who refer those patients to our clinics – have certain expectations, which are the foundation for modern concepts of quality (see "What is quality?," above).

- **Legal obligations:** There are many laws that affect the practice of IVF, and their enforcement is increasingly being achieved via government regulatory agencies – bodies who develop "codes of practice". However, they can also derive from guidelines developed by professional bodies that then become regulations by virtue of being referenced in legislation – an event that might not have been anticipated, and can occur without warning. A good example of this was when the Canadian Fertility and Andrology Society's Guidelines for Therapeutic Donor Insemination were suddenly elevated to the status of regulations by their referencing in the *Processing and Distribution of Semen for Assisted Conception Regulations ("Semen Regulations")* under the authority of the Food and Drugs Act, which led to the Health Canada Directive *Technical Requirements for Therapeutic Donor Insemination*. There is also the whole area of contract law surrounding the provision of services in return for financial considerations.

- **Liability:** Where there are legal obligations and considerations of responsibility, best practice and duty of care, then there are also issues of liability. However, such issues are best left to those qualified in the law, and will not be considered further here!

Implementing TQM

TQM requires a broad approach and skills in many areas, and its successful implementation is utterly dependent upon planning and organization. For example, it has often been said that running an IVF center "requires 10% clinical skills, 30% scientific skills and 60% sheer organization." The important thing here is not to argue over the breakdown of relative professional contributions, but to note the importance attributed to organizational skills.

From a conceptual perspective, implementing TQM requires many things to happen, some of which can be seen as sequential processes, while others will perforce be in parallel. In summary:

- Developing a clear, long-term approach that is integrated with all the organization's other business plans and strategies (e.g. operations, human resources, facility development, information management and technology, fiscal planning).
- Creating a comprehensive collection of policies that address the needs of all areas within the organization. These policies form the skeleton of how TQM will be implemented within the organization and will include goals, objectives, targets, specific projects, and resources. The latter must be developed in full consultation with those individuals who will have the responsibility for translating the policies into achievements.
- Deployment of these policies through all levels of the organization's hierarchy and through all areas of the organization's activities.
- Systems analysis and the integration of quality into all processes at the most fundamental levels.
- Developing prevention-based activities. This includes risk analysis and management and often a cultural shift from fault-finding and blame to recognizing "genuine" mistakes as opportunities for improvement (while not trivializing poor performance or ignoring incompetence).
- Educating everyone in the organization – from the CEO to the "lowest" position – so that they embrace change. Creating a sense of "ownership" is essential in order to achieve "buy-in" from the organization's greatest asset – its people.
- Developing and introducing targeted quality assurance processes so that quality improvement can take place. This is essential for the quality cycle.
- Developing the organization's management and infrastructure to support quality and quality improvement activities. While some new positions will be essential to achieve this (e.g. the quality manager) this should not be seen as a separate part of the organization's management, it must be tightly integrated into the organization's normal business management structure.
- Continuing to pursue standardization, systematization, and simplification of all work instructions, procedures, and systems. Process mapping and systems analysis are essential for this.

The essential steps towards implementing TQM listed above all require focused effort in the following general areas of management:

Leadership

While it is an integral principle that quality is everyone's business, and that everyone must be actively involved, there must be strong leadership from the top. Even though the CEO of a business, or the medical director of an IVF clinic, might not be deeply involved in all the hands-on aspects of implementing a TQM program, they must have some direct participation and provide total support for the process. Such people cannot see themselves as being "special" or have the perspective that quality is "what I employ you all for."

A vital role of senior management is to ensure that the process of implementing TQM does not stall, because this will cause a major loss of faith in the process by the affected personnel – and getting them to buy back in will be far more difficult than it was the first time around.

There is a great deal of excellent advice on how to be a good manager in the *Essential Manager's Manual* (Heller and Hindle, 2003) and we recommend it highly.

Education and training

Everyone in the organization – the directors, managers, and all employees – must be provided with the education to ensure that their general awareness and understanding of quality, its concepts, and the necessary attitudes and skills, is sufficient for them to understand the philosophy of continuous quality improvement and to allow them to participate actively in the process. What might seem like a load of jargon at the outset must become a language of quality that is understood by the entire organization. This requires that it be made relevant to running an IVF center, with explanation given in terms that illustrate its relevance and value.

People must also be taught the tools and techniques that they will need as the process of implementing TQM proceeds. For scientists who have received proper training in scientific method and investigation much of this will be easy, if not second nature. But not everyone will have had the benefit of the highest caliber teachers, and will not, therefore, all be at the same level.

Education and training of its workforce is a large, yet vital, investment that all organizations must be prepared – and able – to take. Without such skills and knowledge it will be difficult for many people to solve problems, and education is a pre-requisite for attitude and behavioral changes (see Chapter 12 for a more detailed discussion of human resources issues). Becoming a "learning organization" is a fundamental principle of accreditation schemes.

Using tools and techniques

In addition to knowing the basic biology and other related scientific disciplines that affect gametes and embryos, effective employment of tools and techniques is necessary for systems analysis, problem solving, technology development, and quality improvement. Without adequate knowledge of such tools and techniques the speed of change, and hence of TQM implementation, will be slowed. In the case of insufficient knowledge, or inadequately widespread knowledge, the entire process could fail.

Involvement and commitment

Employee interest and active participation in quality improvement are vital, not just throughout the period of TQM implementation, but must be a normal part of everyday activities in a "quality" organization. Through this involvement employees develop a sense of "ownership" in their work, which leads to an ongoing sense of commitment to ensuring that everyone, and hence the organization as an entity, does their best. With this increased involvement comes a desire for more active participation and a feeling of satisfaction in the organization's achievements, in other words "buy-in."

Enhanced job satisfaction is very important for employee retention, and also facilitates management. Indeed, along with these sorts of changes, and the seeking of – and listening to – employees' opinions on the organization's activities by managers, comes what many consider to be the greatest benefit of all: increased morale. As a corollary to this closer involvement of employees in the business comes the need for managers to share some of their powers (real or perceived!) and responsibilities. But rather than being the "thin end of the wedge" or "the start of the slippery slope," a good manager will see this, and promote it, as a mechanism for staff coaching/mentoring. The bonus is that this is all achieved with the implicit participation of the staff; there is no need for coercion or for short-term financial or artificial rewards.

As a result of this involvement, there is increased recognition that an organization's employees are its greatest asset – one that will appreciate over time. Concern for, and support of, professional development, as well as providing a career structure, are too often ignored in many industries, including IVF labs. We all know that it takes a long time to properly train a new IVF scientist, yet how many of us have ever tried to put a value on this investment? Helping people realize their potential is rewarding on many levels. Staff development and retention are integral to accreditation schemes and merely reflect one of the most basic business principles: don't allow your competitor to acquire your assets (see Chapter 12 for further discussion of these topics).

Teamwork

Everyone working in IVF knows that it can only be successful if it is based on sound teamwork. It is a multidisciplinary field and while successful outcomes might be achieved if everyone does their job properly, the highest success rates seem to come (usually) from those centers where there is well-defined teamwork – a spirit of community among the staff.

Teams are created for many different reasons, but, as discussed already, creating effective teams is probably the key factor in achieving successful TQM. Teams are a very effective means of maximizing the rate of change in systems because they allow access to the full repertoire of skills of all the members – combining the best features of each while minimizing the impact of any particular individual's weakness. The true strength and potential for achievement of a successful team is not merely the sum of the complementary skills and strengths of its members, a dynamic is created that generates an output that is synergistic, not just additive.

Creating effective teams requires a structured approach, not just a simple process of delegating people based on their apparent availability (remember that the most effective people are usually the busiest), or being the next in line. It involves:

- Analyzing the purpose of the team. Definition of its goals and tasks.
- Knowing the skills and strengths of all available staff, as well as their weaknesses and short-comings.
- Identifying the person who is best-suited to take the lead in the particular task.
- Ensuring that the team membership includes the spectrum of necessary talent.
- Providing the correct reporting structure and necessary external resources.
- Setting an appropriate and adequate timetable for the project.

Beyond recognizable, probably task-orientated or purpose-specific, teams there is also the requirement for everyone to work together. We have already considered this in some depth, and won't labor the point here any further than to say that implementing TQM depends on mutual respect (both professional and personal) and appreciation for everyone in the organization, as well as a recognition that honesty, sincerity, and care, in addition to competence, must be integral to daily work life. There must also be an acceptance that no-one is perfect, and that a mistake is an opportunity for improvement.

Measurement and feedback

In TQM, as in life, you need to be able to measure each task in terms of an output or result. If you can't, then it will seem like some never-ending chore, and you won't have any way of knowing whether you've achieved a goal or not. There has to be an endpoint, as well as a "feel good" factor. We discuss Indicators in detail in Chapter 10, but for the moment it's sufficient to know that you must identify or devise some way of measuring the progress, outcome, or result of any action or process that is undertaken.

An ongoing process

TQM is not a short-term project. It is not "finished" once the initial certification, etc., has been awarded. Like an accreditation scheme, TQM is a never-ending process of continually seeking improvement. In both TQM and accreditation there is a continuum of quality cycle events, although in accreditation the continuum is punctuated by surveys.

Why does TQM fail?

Actually, TQM per se does not fail – but its implementation might. Common causes for an organization not being successful in implementing an effective TQM program include the following problems:

- Insufficient or inappropriate human and/or financial resources.
- Lack of commitment by and/or support from the management ("hollow words").
- Resistance to change, either active or passive (see "Resistance to change," below).
- Insufficient knowledge and/or understanding of what was required.
- Inadequate information management resources and/or systems (includes documentation and data).
- Wrong attitudes or an inappropriate environment (e.g. a culture of fear, fault-finding, blame and retribution, see "The toxic workplace," below).

Resistance to change

This is expressed most commonly by the epithet illustrated in Figure 3.3, but we must also recognize that it is an intrinsic feature of human nature to be frightened of change. But confident, competent people can learn that change is a good thing, that the challenges (and perhaps a little residual fear) that it brings lead to major rewards, not just professional, but personal and financial. Resistance to change can be either passive or active.

Passive resistance to change is best characterized as inertia. How often do you hear the complaint "We don't have enough time!"? Provided that you have established that there are, indeed, sufficient human resources for the

If it ain't broke . . . don't fix it!

Figure 3.3 A common expression of human nature with regard to the perceived need for change.

task or project, then this can be a red flag to identify passive resistance. The individual(s) concerned need to be listened to and then counselled, encouraged, and supported in adapting to the (new) culture of change. If such educational efforts do not work then you might well have to ask whether such people are in the right job, and whether they might find life easier working somewhere else. Unfortunately team building is not always about being supportive and doing positive things, sometimes immovable obstacles need to be removed.

Active resistance is where someone takes positive action to block, undermine or destroy changes that have been introduced. Again, a good manager will be considerate and make every reasonable effort to help the unfortunate person adapt to the modern world, but here the emphasis is definitely on "reasonable."

The textbook by Heller and Hindle (2003) provides a wealth of advice on managing change.

The toxic workplace

If people lack confidence or are insecure in their competence, employment situation or personal life, this insecurity is often displayed in behavior that has been called the "detection-based mentality" (see Figure 3.4). An integral part of TQM is providing support to all staff members to allow them to develop as professionals and rise above such short-comings. However, if the managers (or owners) suffer the same issues themselves, then there is often an abuse of power that leads to a massive escalation of the problem until the organization becomes what has been described as a "toxic workplace" ("*a place where people come to work so they can make enough money so they can leave it*": Jeffrey Pfeffer, cited in Coombs, 2001). By constantly criticizing or disrespecting the staff, these managers feel better able to "control" them and, at the same time, prevent anyone questioning their authority (which is not based on respect) or their competence.

Ann Coombs (2001) gives the example of a tree to describe the effect of a toxic workplace. She explains that while trees are able to withstand storms and drought, if you poison the soil around the tree, the poison will be drawn into the tree through its roots. The poison will collect slowly in the tree, but its effect won't be noticed until the leaves start to turn yellow, and the tree withers and dies, ready to be knocked over by the smallest force. Because of this hidden damage caused by workplace toxicity, she suggests that it is easier to recognize a toxic workplace in retrospect, but gives the following indicators:

- No support for workers from management;
- No support between the workers themselves;
- Lethargy;
- Absenteeism;

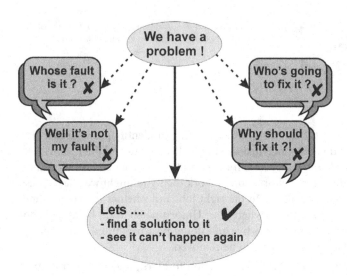

Figure 3.4 An illustration of the "detection-based mentality."

- Verbal and physical intimidation;
- An increased level of complaints;
- Changes in employees' behavior, e.g. loss of confidence or initiative, declining inter-personal relationships, development of turf wars, incidences of "work rage," avoidance of company social functions; and
- A culture of fear.

If you find yourself in a toxic workplace then TQM will never be successful in the long term – although there might be some short-term benefits before everyone gets ground down again. An IVF center that suffers from this syndrome might well be successful in passing an accreditation exercise, but it will never reap the true long-term rewards of everyone's efforts because as soon as the survey is over things will drift back to their previous distasteful state. If the culprit is a manager then hopefully the system will identify him/her and remove this human obstacle from the path towards excellence, but if the source of the problem is the owner then there is only one solution to save your sanity – find a new job! Take your professional skills, and your experience with TQM, to an organization that will value them. Being a bully only works if people accept the bullying.

Quality itself is not the goal

The process of achieving quality is not a self-serving goal, the quality sought has to be useful. Quality must also be real, anyone can attach the word "quality" to their activities or systems, but unless there is true commitment and achievement the supposed quality program will not survive. Quality management cannot stand alone, it has to be integrated into all levels of the organization's operations and embraced on a daily basis.

Common roots of quality management philosophies

Any internet search on quality management will reveal a range of philosophies beyond the "generic" TQM philosophy – but how different are they in reality?

WE Deming

It is generally accepted that TQM started with the work of the American statistician W (William) Edwards Deming (1900–1993). While Deming was widely credited with improving industrial production in the USA during World War II, it was his work in post-war Japan, teaching industry management about improved design, product quality, and testing – and hence sales and service – for which he is best known. Early in his career Deming was profoundly influenced by the work of Shewhart (see below), a fellow statistician then working for Bell Telephone Laboratories, who created the concepts of statistical control of processes. Deming's book *Out of the Crisis* (1986) is an excellent overview of his life and work, and is the basis for the remainder of this section.

Deming's overall philosophy has been summarized in equation form showing how quality tends to increase and costs fall over time:

Quality = Results of work efforts / Total costs

The following truisms stem from this:

- Productivity increases as quality improves because there is less re-work and not so much waste.
- Defects that get into the hands of customers cost market share, and cost workers their jobs.
- Low quality means high cost because someone gets paid for both making and correcting defects.
- Most gains in productivity must come from improving the system, improvements to help people work smarter, not harder.

The following conceptualizations show Deming's profound insightfulness and reveals his true role as one of the most important industrial figures of the twentieth century, based on the need to understand a system (via his "System of Profound Knowledge," see below) before being able to change it ("transformation" in Deming's parlance), and the recognition that the individual is the key first step to achieving change via a discontinuous process that embraces every aspect of the organization. Once "transformed" an individual will:

- Set an example;
- Be a good listener (without compromising oneself);
- Continually teach others; and
- Help others leave behind their current practices and beliefs, allowing them to move into the new philosophy without feeling guilty about the past.

These are still, today, the key principles in managing change in any organization.

Deming's System of Profound Knowledge

1. Appreciation of a system: the need to understand the overall processes involving suppliers, producers and customers of goods and services.
2. Knowledge of variation: the range and causes of variation in quality, and the use of statistical sampling in measurements.
3. Theory of knowledge: the concepts explaining knowledge, and the limits of what can be known.
4. Knowledge of psychology: concepts explaining and permitting understanding of human nature.

Deming's 14 Points

In *Out of the Crisis*, Deming proposed 14 key principles for managing the transformation of business effectiveness:

1. Create constancy of purpose towards improvement of products and services.
2. Adopt the new philosophy; managers must become leaders. See Chapter 12.
3. Cease dependence on inspection to achieve quality; build quality into the product in the first place.
4. Do not award business based simply on price, instead minimize total cost by consolidating suppliers with whom you have long-term relationships based on loyalty and trust.
5. Constantly improve the system of production and service: improve quality while minimizing costs.
6. Institute training on the job.
7. Institute leadership. (The aim of supervision should be to help people and technology do a better job; this includes management as well as production workers.)
8. Drive out fear so that everyone can work effectively; this can only benefit the organization.
9. Break down barriers between departments.
10. Eliminate slogans, exhortations, even target goals, etc., aimed at the work force – the majority of the root causes of problems are inherent to the system, and hence beyond the power of the workforce to change.
11. Eliminate work standards (quotas) and "management by objectives," instead substitute Leadership. (If the system is stable there is no need to specify a goal, you will get what the system produces.)
12. Remove barriers that rob production workers of their right to pride of workmanship, and change the responsibility of supervisors from quantity to quality. Remove barriers that rob managers and designers (including engineers) of their right to pride of workmanship: abolish automatic annual or other merit rewards that are based on management by objective.
13. Institute a vigorous program of education and self-improvement for everyone within the organization.
14. Put everyone in the organization to work on accomplishing the transformation.

Deming's Seven Deadly Diseases

These concepts can be applied far beyond manufacturing or service industries – just consider them in regard to everyday life, or politics:

1. Lack of constancy of purpose. Long-term planning is essential to stay in business, it provides for secure management and security of employment.
2. Emphasis on short-term profits. Chasing increases in quarterly production or sales figures, or dividends, undermines quality and productivity.
3. Evaluation by performance, merit rating, or annual reviews of performance. These can be devastating, through destroying teamwork, nurturing rivalry, and leading to individuals experiencing fear, bitterness and despondency; they also promote mobility of management.
4. Mobility of management. Job-hopping managers never understand the companies they work for, and are never around long enough to follow through on long-term changes

that are essential for improved quality and productivity. Hopefully this is not readily apparent in the ART field.

5. Running a company on visible figures alone. The most important figures are unknown and unknowable, e.g. the multiplier effect of satisfied customers.
6. Excessive medical costs (considered a US-specific problem).
7. Excessive costs of warranty, fuelled by lawyers who work for contingency fees. While this was also considered a US-specific problem, it is fast becoming a global issue.

In the modern world one might also consider adding the disease of excessive regulatory costs, especially those arising out of "user pays" or "cost recovery" governmental programs.

It is evident that Deming created the foundation for modern quality management, and his concepts and philosophies underpin everything that we shall consider in this book.

WA Shewhart

Walter Andrew Shewhart (1891–1967) was an American physicist, engineer, and statistician, and is often described as the father of statistical quality control. His work with Bell Telephone and Western Electric Company was based on improving the reliability of telephone transmission systems, since much of the equipment was buried underground, and hence needed to be dependable. Industrial quality after World War I was limited to the inspection of finished products and the rejection of defective items. But in 1924 Shewhart proposed the control chart (see Chapter 6), and process quality control was born. His work has been summarized in the book *Statistical Method from the Viewpoint of Quality Control* (1939, republished 1986).

Shewhart's basic principle was that bringing a production process into a state of statistical control, where there is only a chance-cause variation, and then keeping it in control, is necessary to predict future output and manage a process economically. He formulated the statistical concept of tolerance intervals, and proposed two extremely important rules for presenting data:

• Data have no meaning apart from their context.
• Data contain both signal and noise; to be able to extract information from data one must separate the signal from the noise.

Shewhart's world involved measurements of physical processes, which never produce a Gaussian "normal distribution" of results. In biological systems, we need to add the principle of uncertainty of measurement (see Chapter 6) to Shewhart's rules to fully understand the quality of data, and the limitations that might exist in their interpretation. Remember:

Data ≠ Information ≠ Knowledge ≠ Understanding

Biological systems require more careful analysis to permit the derivation and synthesis of ideas, and their integration into the real-world framework. This often involves successive generations standing on the shoulders of the giants of preceding generations. After all, it is only 40 years ago that Bob Edwards, Alan Trounson, and Alex Lopata, working with their clinical collaborators, Patrick Steptoe, Carl Wood, and Ian Johnston, were still working to make clinical IVF a reality.

A brief overview of quality frameworks

While we have embraced the generic framework of TQM (popularized in the 1980s) for many years, readers will no doubt have heard of a variety of business quality management strategies such as "Six Sigma," "Kaizen", and "Lean." There are numerous books published on these systems, and space precludes a detailed discussion of their operational processes, strengths, and weaknesses here. However, there are many commonalities, both among them and with TQM, as well as a few limitations in regard to the IVF laboratory. Some books that integrate many of these aspects include George *et al.* (2005), and Graban and Swartz (2014).

Six Sigma

This business strategy, often referred to by its abbreviation "6σ," was originally developed by Motorola USA in 1981. The name originated from statistical modeling terminology, sigma being an abbreviation for the standard deviation, and is founded on the principle of achieving a defect rate of just 3.4 per million (i.e. 99.99966% correct, although this is an inherently arbitrary target). A "defect" is defined as any process output that does not meet customer specifications, or that could lead to creating an output that does not meet customer specifications. Immediately one can see that these goals are generically similar to those of any quality/risk management system.

However, the target of having a process whose mean performance value is at least six standard deviations from the nearest specification limit – so that almost no product item will fail to meet those specifications – does have limitations. For example, one generalization is that processes often do not perform as well in the long term as they do in the short term, perhaps reflecting the inability of the process (or its machinery or operators) to maintain its original very high engineering specifications when operating under everyday conditions. This is the basis for an in-built 1.5 SD "buffer" (since, in fact, a 3.4-per-million failure rate is achieved at only 4.5 SD from the mean value in a Normally distributed dataset). At least one statistician has described this inherent provision for an arbitrary 1.5σ shift as "goofy."

While Six Sigma might be well suited to an engineering-based manufacturing process, its suitability for an "industry" such as IVF, which is based on biological processes, is likely to be fraught with difficulties. Moreover, assisted conception treatment is a human-resource-driven healthcare process that must be flexible and readily adaptable according to each couple's etiology and needs. So, although Six Sigma has been applied across many industries (albeit with some controversy), its applicability in IVF clearly has severe limitations.

Six Sigma seeks to improve process quality by identifying and removing the causes of defects (errors) in process output(s). The goal is to minimize variability in manufacturing or business processes using a relatively rigid framework of quality management methods, especially statistical process control, through the efforts of a special infrastructure of Six Sigma methodology experts within the organization. Managing a project according to 6σ principles follows one of two five-step methodologies, both inspired by Deming's plan, do, check, act (PDCA) cycle (see Chapter 7), which have been summarized in Table 3.1. The general equivalence of DMAIC and DMADV to root cause analysis and failure modes and effects analysis, respectively, should be apparent.

Within Six Sigma the creation of an infrastructure of experts (professionals specialized in quality management functions) was seen as a key innovation, but it has also been criticized for its creation of a population of "itinerant change agents," change management experts who themselves are the product of an industry of training and certification. The formalized role of

Table 3.1 Comparison of the two five-step methodologies for project management according to Six Sigma principles

DMAIC	DMADV
For improving an existing process	For designing a new product or process (also sometimes called "DFSS" or "Design for Six Sigma").
Define the problem, the purpose of the process (the "customer voice"), the project goals, as precisely as possible.	Define design goals that are consistent with customer expectations, and within the enterprise strategy.
Measure key aspects of the current process, collect relevant data ("Indicators").	Measure (after identifying) characteristics that are "critical to quality" ("CTQs," which can be seen as equivalent to "Indicators") in terms of product capabilities, production process capabilities, and risks.
Analyze the data to investigate and verify cause-and-effect relationships (i.e. undertake a root cause analysis).	Analyze to develop and design alternatives and select the best design based on its capability to match a high-level design concept (the "ideal").
Improve or optimize the current process; in manufacturing this might involve the creation of a new, "future state" process that can be run on a pilot basis.	Design details, optimize the design, and plan for design verification (this phase might require the production of prototypes or use simulations).
Control the future state process to verify that any deviations from the target have been corrected. Implement control systems (e.g. process control using Shewhart Charts of appropriate Indicators) to continuously monitor the process.	Verify the design, set up pilot runs, implement the production process; the task is complete only when the process has been handed over to its owner(s).

the Six Sigma experts as "rulers" of change and quality management can stifle creativity, perhaps by discouraging or even blocking innovations that (would have) come from "below." And blind adherence to DMAIC rules could lead to merely serial incremental innovations rather than a creative re-imagining of a process brought about through review by fresh eyes or someone who stands back and says "what if?" (a loss of blue sky thinking).

While manufacturing industries might all have very similar control issues and possible solutions, the qualities required in a quality manager for an IVF lab (more properly an IVF clinic) are very different – and the needs of the gametes and embryos, and how these impact patient management, are very different from almost every other area of healthcare. Our experience has been that quality and risk management within the IVF lab/clinic is really only successful when everyone is actively involved in all aspects of the QMS; the quality manager has an important role, but ideally as a "ring master," rather than as a "fat controller" (apologies to Thomas The Tank Engine fans!).

Kaizen

Kaizen is a Japanese word meaning "improvement" or "change for the better," and in the business sense refers to the philosophy or practices that focus on continuous quality improvement – in manufacturing, engineering, business processes, or management.

Workplace Kaizen includes all activities that seek to or support continuous functional improvement, it involves everyone, from the CEO to janitorial staff, as well as certain external stakeholders, and includes support services (e.g. purchasing, logistics) that cross organizational boundaries and influence the supply chain. By standardizing and improving processes and systems, Kaizen seeks to eliminate waste – and hence has many close similarities with lean manufacturing (see below). The key elements of Kaizen are usually stated as quality, effort, involvement of all staff, willingness to change, and communication – essentially the same as TQM. Kaizen also mirrors TQM through its five main elements of teamwork, personal discipline, improved morale, quality circles (i.e. PDCA Cycles), and suggestions for improvement.

However, the purpose of Kaizen goes beyond simply improving manufacturing productivity; adherence to the principles of Kaizen also humanizes the workplace, and can therefore be seen as highly appropriate for the human resource-intensive systems of the IVF lab or clinic. Other benefits of Kaizen include the elimination of overly hard work (see also "muri" in the section on Lean, below), teaching staff how to apply the scientific method to analyze and improve their work tasks, and how to identify – and eliminate – waste within systems. Notwithstanding these clear benefits, overzealous application of Kaizen can also be detrimental. For example, repeated cost-cutting measures could be at the expense of fair labor practices, reduced component quality, and hence decreased quality of the final product. An excellent consideration of the application of Kaizen in healthcare has recently been published (Graben and Swartz, 2014), considering not just its strengths and practical aspects of implementation, but also illustrating its weaknesses and possible pitfalls.

Kaizen is probably best known in regard to the Toyota Production System, with which it has been seen as almost synonymous. At Toyota, production personnel are expected to stop the line in case of an abnormality, and then work with their supervisor to suggest an improvement using Kaizen tools. A focused bout of Kaizen activity is often referred to as a "Kaizen blitz," and can give rise to further blitzes as the focus widens or deepens. The Toyota Production System also gave us the concept of "just-in-time" (JIT), seeking to optimize "flow" with minimal inventory (Deming, 1986). But anyone who has managed an IVF lab knows that JIT is simply impossible within the responsible provision of IVF treatment in a world where materials supply is unreliable and unpredictable. Many IVF labs operate a stock control system that always maintains at least two or three months of essential supplies, and accreditation schemes expect this sort of risk management.

Unfortunately, other major criticisms of Kaizen have also come out of the Toyota Production System, including death from overwork stemming from unpaid, "voluntary" quality control meetings held after regular work hours. Healthcare has also provided criticism of Kaizen in situations where direct care providers such as nurses have gone on strike following Kaizen-driven streamlining procedures that have been used to reduce staff: patient ratios to reduce costs, but failing to recognize that medical procedure times and the provision of patient-centered care cannot always be standardized.

So while Kaizen principles have clear applicability in the IVF lab or clinic, the implementation of change must recognize the real-world aspects of each process, and of the system as a whole – especially in the private sector, where patient expectations for their standard of care are higher. Basically, the entire clinic must respect the patients throughout their treatment experience, with the lab also focusing on respecting the physiology of their gametes and embryos.

Lean

The commonly used term "Lean" derives from "lean manufacturing," "lean production" or "lean enterprise," and refers to a production practice that considers the expenditure of resources for any purpose other than the creation of value for the end customer to be wasteful, and thus a target for elimination. Hence Lean works from the "market-in" perspective, with "value" being defined as something a customer would be willing to pay for: as waste is eliminated quality improves, while production time and costs are reduced.

Lean is centered on preserving or improving value with less (most often less work), and is inherent within Kaizen. Indeed, the philosophy of lean manufacturing is largely based on the Toyota Production System (see above), and the term "lean" was only applied to it in the 1990s, although the term was first coined in 1988 (Krafcik, 1988).

A Lean process is achieved through the reduction of three general types of waste, often referred to by their Japanese terms:

1. *Muda*, or non-value-adding work;
2. *Muri*, or overburden (e.g. pushing a person or machine beyond their natural limits); and
3. *Mura*, or unevenness (achieved through improving the flow or smoothness of work).

Linking them within a Lean framework is quite simple:

1. *Muri* focuses on process preparation of planning, avoiding unnecessary work when the process is first designed [akin to failure modes and effects analysis];
2. *Mura* focuses on how the design is implemented, including the elimination of fluctuations caused by scheduling or other variable levels of operation (e.g. volume, even quality); and
3. *Muda* is then discovered after the process is in place, and dealt with reactively [as per root cause analysis].

Types of waste

The Toyota Production System considered seven "muda" or sources of waste:

1. Transport or transit (moving things that are not actually required to perform the process);
2. Inventory (all components, work-in-progress, and unused finished product);
3. Motion (people or equipment moving more than is necessary to perform the process);
4. Waiting (delays between process steps, interruptions due to shift changes, etc.);
5. Overproduction (production ahead of demand);
6. Overprocessing (resulting from poor product or process design that causes unnecessary activity); and
7. Defects (actual wastage, as well as the effort expended in inspecting for and fixing defects).

Since the original elaboration of the Toyota Production System, other sources of waste have also been defined:

8. Manufacturing goods or services that do not meet customer demand or expectations;
9. Waste of unused human talent, identified in Six Sigma as under-utilizing capabilities, as well as delegating tasks with inadequate training;

10. Space (since space costs money for construction, rental, heating/cooling, cleaning, etc.);
11. Working to the wrong or no metrics (a process cannot be monitored, and hence cannot be improved, if it is not being measured);
12. Not utilizing a complete worker by not allowing them to contribute ideas and suggestions; and
13. Improper use of computers (insufficient workstations or logons, not having the proper software and/or not having adequate training on how to use software, as well as lost ["stolen"?] time spent surfing the web or playing games).

For example, Kaizen's just-in-time philosophy reduces inventory and facilitates production up-scaling, it also saves on storage space for all the raw materials or components (Toyota enjoyed an estimated 30% space saving compared with comparable US automobile manufacturers: Deming, 1986).

Lean aims to make a work process simple enough for its operators to understand, perform, and manage, and its implementation focuses on getting the right things to the right place at the right time in the right quantity to achieve perfect work flow (while both minimizing waste and being flexible and able to change). Simple, right? But if we don't focus on some magic term ("lean"), and instead simply employ process mapping and analysis, combining prospective FMEAs with retrospective RCAs as required, then Lean is only another way of applying TQM principles.

Illustrating Lean

In addition to the better known tools such as process maps and the PDCA cycle, Lean makes extensive use of visual tools to illustrate and analyze the process under consideration. An excellent software suite for these purposes is SmartDraw (San Diego, CA, USA), which provides many easy to work with templates.

Value stream maps are used to analyze and design the flow of processes, primarily information and materials flows, needed to bring a product or service to the customer. Like more standard flow charts, value stream mapping is quite formalized, employing standard symbols to represent items and processes. Originally conceived by Henry Ford in the 1920s, value stream maps are a core element of the Toyota Production System, and are a recognized tool used in Six Sigma methodologies.

A standardized value stream map format has the value-adding steps drawn across the center of the map and the non-value-adding steps represented in vertical lines at right angles to the value stream, easily separating the "waste" steps from the value stream activities. Each vertical line can be seen as the "story" of a person or workstation, while the horizontal line represents the overall process.

Fishbone or *cause-and-effect diagrams* (sometimes referred to as Ishikawa diagrams, see Figure 3.5) are useful for brainstorming sessions, allowing users to drill down into a process to identify where problems are occurring. They are commonly employed in product design and quality defect prevention, to identify potential factors causing an overall effect. Within the diagram, causes are typically grouped into six major categories to identify these factors: People (anyone involved with the process); Methods (how the process is performed and the specific requirements for doing it, e.g. policies, procedures, rules, regulations); Machines (any equipment, computers, tools, etc., required to perform the process); Materials (all raw materials, components, pens, paper, etc., used within the process); Measurements (any data generated from the process that can be used to evaluate its quality); and Environment (all

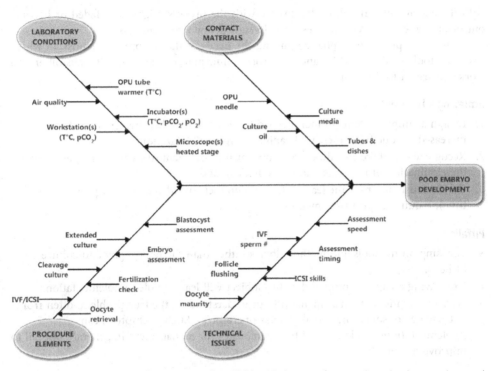

Figure 3.5 A simple example of a cause-and-effect ("fishbone") diagram of poor embryo development (prepared using a template from SmartDraw, San Diego, CA, USA).

the conditions within which the process operates). An IDEF0 process map can be seen as a combination of process map and fishbone diagram.

Spaghetti diagrams are used to detail the actual physical flow and distances involved in a work process. They are most often used to illustrate a system's inefficiency, and enable a critical analysis of the movement of material or people within the workspace with the goal of eliminating transit waste. However, a spaghetti diagram can also be used to illustrate an efficient and ergonomic lab design, for instance (see Chapter 7).

Kanban boards are a simple, yet powerful tool to visualize workflow, allowing staff to focus on a limited number of more important tasks. The simplest Kanban board consists of just three columns: "to-do," "in progress," and "done." By limiting work in progress the identification of bottlenecks will be facilitated.

SIPOC (suppliers, inputs, process, outputs, and customers) is a commonly used Six Sigma and Lean process improvement tool that summarizes the inputs and outputs of the process in tabular form, using a column for each component of the acronym. In a SIPOC analysis the focus is on capturing the inputs and outputs rather than the individual steps in the process. Suppliers and customers can be internal or external to the organization that performs the process, and inputs and outputs can be materials, services, or information.

A SIPOC analysis is often presented at the outset of a process improvement effort (e.g. the "define" phase of the Six Sigma DMAIC process, or a Kaizen event). Depending on the audience, a SIPOC table can serve as an overview of the process for staff who are unfamiliar with it, re-acquaint staff whose familiarity with the process might have faded or become out-of-date due to process changes, or help staff define a new process.

Some users prefer to emphasize putting the needs of the customer foremost, in which cases the tool is called COPIS, and the process information starts with the customer and works upstream to the supplier.

Achieving a Lean system

1. Design a simple system (in manufacturing: decreased cycle time, less inventory, increased productivity, increased capital equipment utilization);
2. Recognize that there will always be room for improvement (the core principle of Lean is the elimination of non-value-added activities); and
3. Continuously improve the lean system design (achieve incremental improvements over time); requires appropriate metrics.

Pitfalls

- Focusing on the tools and methodologies rather than the philosophy and culture of Lean.
- Not having adequate command of the subject will lead to failed implementation.
- Decisions made by management without understanding the true problem, often from not having consulted the actual process operator(s). Such attempted Lean implementations can look good to the manager (or management in general), but fail to improve the situation.

Chapter

4

What is risk?

Reducing medical errors and enhancing patient and staff safety is a prime focus in modern medicine. But what is "risk"?

Put simply, a risk is any uncertainty about a future event that might threaten an organization's ability to accomplish its mission. It is the chance of something happening that will have a negative impact on an organization's objectives. In particular, risk is the possibility of suffering "loss": loss of quality of outcome, loss of professional regard or profile, loss of referrals, loss of patient/staff health (or even loss of life), loss of profitability, loss of success. It is said that failure is a key part of learning, and that in business risk and opportunity often go hand-in-hand, with risk per se not only being not bad, but even essential to progress. Clearly such a perception of risk "as a good thing" is not acceptable in IVF centers.

Continued developments in reproductive biomedicine, combined with heightened regulatory requirements, have led to more, unexpected, and often complex, risk issues for IVF centers. It is now more important than ever to be proactive in identifying risk and taking appropriate preventative measures, hence IVF centers must embrace risk analysis and risk minimization. Together, these constitute risk management, which is an integral part of total quality management or "TQM" (see Chapter 3) and any ISO 9000 family-compliant quality system or laboratory accreditation scheme. The last two decades have seen much effort expended on "clinical governance," which is a process essentially synonymous with TQM for medical practice, and a lot of attention has been focused on iatrogenic illness (Sharpe and Faden, 1998). For a review of risk management in IVF from the clinical perspective, see the article by Richard Kennedy (Kennedy, 2004).

Risk management was originally an engineering discipline dealing with the possibility that some future event might cause harm. It includes strategies and techniques for recognizing and confronting any such threat and provides a disciplined environment for proactive decision-making for the purpose of:

- Assessing on a continuous basis what can go wrong;
- Determining which risks need to be dealt with; and
- Implementing strategies to deal with these risks.

Risk management can summarized as asking – and answering – three basic questions:

1. "What can go wrong?";
2. "What will we do?" (both to prevent the harm from occurring and in the aftermath of an incident); and
3. "If something happens, how will we resolve it, put things right and/or pay for it?"

A widely used standard for managing risk (e.g. by the UK National Health Service) in the early 2000s was the Australia and New Zealand Standard "Risk Management" AS/NZS4360:2004, but it has been superseded by AS/NZS ISO 31000:2009, which is a joint Australia/New Zealand adoption of ISO 31000:2009 *Risk Management – Principles and Guidelines.*

An excellent example of how a corporation might deal with potential future risk that was well-known in ART labs was the prohibition of using Percoll for any clinical application by its manufacturer, Pharmacia Biotech AB of Uppsala, Sweden, effective January 1, 1997 (Mortimer, 2000). Percoll is a general-purpose laboratory reagent not manufactured to the standards required for a medical device. To do so would have made it prohibitively expensive for the vast majority of its users, who employed it for research purposes only – as illustrated by the higher cost of replacement products that are manufactured and registered as medical devices, e.g. PureSperm (Nidacon International, AB, Göteborg, Sweden).

But the value of an effective risk management program is not limited just to reducing the economic impacts of indemnity (insurance) and claims (litigation). Fears of criminal prosecution within the biomedical community are not without foundation, and the economic impact of effective risk management should also be measured by the development of goodwill and the increased level of satisfaction experienced by everyone involved (patients, staff, and management). Because patient satisfaction is closely associated with quality, a successful risk management program is also a powerful marketing tool. Managers in non-healthcare industries do not rely on price alone to sell their products (either goods or services) to customers, and modern-thinking employers and employees want to know about safety. This all adds up to a better quality service, and in the field of assisted conception, that is what the increasingly better-educated and more sophisticated patients and referrers (an IVF center's customers) are looking for.

A major benefit of an effective risk management program, in which risks are continuously identified, analyzed, and minimized, mitigated or eliminated, is that problems are prevented before they occur: there is a cultural shift from "fire-fighting" and "crisis management" to proactive decision-making and planning. Anticipating what might go wrong becomes inherent in everyday operations. While implementing risk management is no "magic bullet" – it does not guarantee success (because there are many aspects to achieving success in an IVF center) – but it does improve decision-making, help avoid surprises, and improve the chances of succeeding.

The consequences of *not* pursuing risk management are that:

- More resources will be expended to correct problems that could have been avoided;
- Catastrophic problems will occur without warning;
- There will be no ability to respond rapidly to such "surprises" and recovery will be very difficult and/or costly, or even impossible;
- Decisions will be made with incomplete information or inadequate knowledge of their possible future consequences;
- The overall probability of success will be reduced; and
- The organization will always be in a state of crisis.

Identifying "high-risk" IVF laboratories

IVF is an area of rapidly advancing technology, meaning that continual training and proficiency testing are imperative. But these tactics in isolation will not prevent the type of problems that keep appearing in the mass media, and we must recognize that the overall environment in which people work can either support or obstruct both technical training and improvements in operational systems. Is it possible for a hospital or fertility center to identify whether their IVF laboratory is at particular risk for adverse events, especially of the "high profile" kind? From experience, the following are the most likely areas where such risk factors might be identified (but it must be stressed that this is by no means an exhaustive risk analysis of an IVF Lab).

Staffing issues

- *Insufficient staff.* A recent UK-based workload analysis revealed that over 70% of IVF labs there are understaffed (Harbottle, 2003). This study confirmed our own earlier (unpublished) calculations that in an IVF laboratory operating to established quality standards, one full-time embryologist is required for each 125 stimulated treatment cycles per annum.
- *Overworking.* In order to perform all aspects of their jobs accurately and reliably, with the lowest possible risk of making mistakes, embryologists must be alert and not distracted by tiredness. Any circumstances that contribute to overtiredness or exhaustion represent serious risk factors. Staffing levels should reflect the maximum caseload – some slack must be available within the system so that staff are not constantly working at their maximum capacity. Risk factors might include regularly working more than 48 hours per week or more than six consecutive days without at least one full day's rest.
- *Inexperienced staff.* Even with effective training programs, a high staff turnover increases the number of people who are less sure of the laboratory's systems, standard operating procedures (SOPs), and usual practices. Laboratories that have a higher proportion of relatively inexperienced embryologists will be less equipped to recognize and deal with operational problems as they arise.
- *Poorly trained staff.* Comprehensive, formal programs are essential not only for training all embryologists in new techniques and procedures (i.e. novices and more junior staff), but also for the orientation, and re-training as necessary, of embryologists coming from other laboratories. If someone unintentionally fails to complete all aspects of their assigned tasks then this is an expression of inadequate or incomplete training, and should be easily remedied.
- *Not accepting professional responsibility.* This occurs when one or more members of a team do not take enough care to ensure that they have performed – and completed – all the tasks that were assigned to them. This can be either intentional or unintentional (see above), but in both cases is unprofessional. The intentional omission of parts of one's job can only continue without jeopardizing outcomes if there are others who take the time (and/or are prepared to make the time) to ensure that the whole process is completed: in effect they are the "safety net." All professionals must be prepared to work without a safety net; if someone cannot do this then (s)he should not be working in an IVF lab or, indeed, an IVF clinic.

Resource issues

- *The need for slack.* Slack must be present in any organization to allow not only for the differential between the average and busiest activity levels, but also to cope with "unpredictable" events such as an influenza epidemic. An allowance for slack time is essential for an organization to evolve (DeMarco, 2001).

- *Inadequate resources.* Centers that insist on running with the minimum possible resources (physical, human, or financial) will be at greater risk. There must be sufficient capacity in critical equipment to deal with the busiest of times: e.g. for those labs still using "big-box" incubators, having adequate incubator space so incubator doors are not opened too often, and for labs using incubation systems such as the large-capacity G185 bench-top incubator from K-Systems (or perhaps an Embryoscope), having adequate spare capacity for when an incubator needs servicing or malfunctions.

- *Equipment failure.* All equipment must be included in a preventative maintenance program and all "mission critical" equipment, such as cryostorage tanks, incubators, CO_2 supply, liquid nitrogen supply must be monitored at least routinely (e.g. daily). In addition, there should be an out-of-hours alarm system that can call or page a list of contact persons, any of whom is capable of resolving the issue. More advanced labs are now installing real-time monitoring systems (Mortimer and Di Berardino, 2008), such as the Planer *ReAssure* system (also see Chapter 11).

- *Power failure.* Provisions must be in place to ensure the continuity of electrical power to critical equipment. Items sensitive to power fluctuations need to be protected by a line conditioner or, better, an uninterruptible power supply or "UPS."

Organizational issues

- *Not double-checking.* Every time that something is labelled, or material (i.e. gametes or embryos) is moved from one container to another, identity checks must be followed strictly and verified either by a competent witness or some valid technological solution. In the UK, the HFEA introduced a requirement for "double-witnessing" of all such events in October 2002 (see Brison *et al.*, 2004), and an increasing number of laboratories are installing electronic witnessing technology (Thornhill *et al.*, 2013; also see Chapter 9).

- *Inadequate SOPs.* Incomplete, or poorly written, SOPs create opportunities for embryologists to make mistakes.

- *Omissions.* Lack of: (i) a comprehensive, documented system of notifications, and (ii) task lists to ensure that the laboratory staff know exactly what has to be done each day, will increase the risk of things "falling through the cracks" and critical tasks being forgotten.

- *Unauthorized "improvements" in methods.* All staff must follow the laboratory's SOPs exactly. Any changes to documented SOPs must be authorized by the lab director to ensure that the changes would not be detrimental. Introduction of variations, short-cuts, or perceived "improvements" without authorization should be a disciplinary offence, because of the enormous increase in risk.

Risk management issues

- *Poor documentation.* Great care must be taken when completing all documentation (and everything must be documented) to ensure that all records (laboratory, medical, and government) are complete and accurate. For example, a center that makes repeated mistakes in its submissions of data to an external regulatory agency could be considered suspect in its ability to complete its own paperwork. Other indicators of carelessness or lack of attention to detail (i.e. risk) include personnel not being aware of patients' appointments/procedures/management plan, mistakes in patient accounts, telephone calls being made to the wrong patient, etc.

- *Unrecognized incidents.* Unless a comprehensive system of Incident Reports (in ISO parlance "non-conformity reports") for all adverse events is in place, enforced, and employed constructively, many mistakes will never be recognized or remembered. In this context, an "adverse event" can be defined as any event that potentially or actually affects staff safety, patient safety, or the provision of treatment according to the patient's care plan or the expected outcome of their treatment.

- *Use of non-approved products or devices.* Some IVF centers use products or devices that are either intended for veterinary use or that have not been approved for medical use by the appropriate regulatory authorities, e.g. The Food and Drug Administration in the USA, CE marking in Europe,[2] etc. A common example of this is the Tomcat catheter, a veterinary product that is still used even today in some centers for intra-uterine insemination and even embryo transfer. Studies reported at conferences, and in peer-reviewed journals have clearly demonstrated the detrimental effect of this catheter when used for embryo transfer (see Chapter 11). Consequently, not only is such usage a significant risk factor for decreased success rates, but it must also be considered a risk in terms of potential liability.

Disaster planning

On a larger scale, risk management also includes "disaster planning," four examples of which are summarized here.

> **Earthquake preparedness.** Obviously the consequence of an earthquake could be catastrophic, possibly resulting in the loss of multiple lives and potentially in the total destruction of the facility. If an IVF center is located in, say, the San Francisco area, then the risk level is "likely," and clearly disaster planning must be undertaken. Obviously nothing can be done to reduce the likelihood, since an earthquake is a natural disaster, but the center's disaster plan must take all reasonable steps to mitigate the potential impact of an earthquake upon staff and patients, the embryos in culture, and the contents of the cryobank. However, for a center located in a historically geologically stable part of the world, the earthquake risk would be rated as "very unlikely," and hence would not warrant serious attention.
>
> **Possible meteor strike.** Again the consequence of such a natural disaster would be rated as "catastrophic," but the likelihood must surely be considered to be "very unlikely," meaning that such an event need not be included in a center's disaster planning.
>
> **Anthrax bioterrorism.** Although this issue was, hopefully, a historical anachronism, the October 2001 anthrax attacks via mail in the USA caused greatly heightened awareness of terrorist threats, and planning for risks such as this was undertaken by very many US and Canadian IVF centers. Certainly if an IVF center is located in an area where there is even a

---

[2] Conformance with the EUTCD expects, essentially, that non-CE-marked products should not be used if a CE-marked product is available.

small likelihood of terrorist attack, then provision for coping with any foreseeable types of attacks must be included in the center's disaster planning.

Climate change. Numerous extreme meteorological events over the past year or so have not only demonstrated the truly awesome power of nature, but are eloquent evidence of the reality of climate change. Consequently, practical planning for disasters that can arise as a result of extreme weather must become routine in any area that has experienced such events. Severe flooding, hurricanes, tornados, severe winter storm, and extreme heat waves, and the not just possible resulting bushfires, but also frequent – even sustained – power outages due to shortage of supply, have affected many IVF centers around the world and such climatic risks should probably be seen as the "new norm."

Tools for risk management

There are two main tools used in risk management, one proactive, the other reactive. The proactive tool is called failure modes and effects analysis or "FMEA," and the reactive tool is root cause analysis or "RCA" (see Chapter 7). While FMEA works towards the prevention of risk, RCA is used to deal with actual adverse events and troubleshooting. Because both tools are based upon analyzing systems and processes, understanding the concepts and principles of process mapping is pre-requisite to effective risk management (see Chapter 5). Most risk assessment exercises will generate a *risk matrix*, which is also considered in Chapter 7.

Risk perception and communication

Understanding people's perception and acceptance of risk is a major branch of cognitive psychology, and far too extensive an area to cover in any detail in the present volume. However, from a scientist's perspective, risk communication is a balance between the two fundamental ways in which humans perceive risk: analytically and experientially (Slovik *et al.*, 2004).

The *analytic* or *rational system* is a slow, intensive process that uses algorithms and rules, including probability theory, logic, and risk assessment, and requires conscious control. Being based on images and associations that are linked by experience to emotion and affect (the sense of "good" or "bad"), the *experiential system* is fast, and essentially intuitive. It is largely inaccessible to conscious awareness, and is the most natural way in which people respond to risk. The two systems are not alternatives. but operate inter-dependently: rational decision-making requires their proper integration.

Risk perception

Risk can be considered as existing in three forms:

• Risk that is perceived directly;
• Risk that is perceived through science; and
• Virtual risk.

The interplay between the three forms of risk within the analytic and experiential systems can be summarized as shown in Figure 4.1.

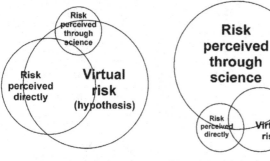

Risk Perception Paradigms

Rational or Analytical System

Experiential System (Reality?)

Figure 4.1 Simplified illustration of the interplay between the three forms of risk within the analytic and experiential paradigms.

How someone behaves in regard to risk can be seen as a balancing act between four forces:

- The value of reward from an action;
- The individual's propensity towards taking risk;
- The individual's perception of danger; and
- The fear of accidents.

Different social cultures and environments will create and modify filters between reward and risk-taking, and between perceived danger and fear of accidents. The end result is a balance of behavior that "defines" the individual. As over-simplifications, while medical and scientific staff are generally biased towards the analytic system, patients – and the public at large – typically employ more experiential approaches towards risk; and part of the consultation and counselling processes during ART treatment should endeavor to help patients comprehend the risks of treatment more analytically. Indeed, without effective risk communication, establishing informed consent is impossible.

Risk communication scales

A variety of "scales" have been described to facilitate risk communication to non-expert people. Most of them are based on increasing order of magnitude (i.e. they are logarithmic in nature) and are often likened to "Richter Scales" for risks (Calman and Royston, 1997).

The *Calman Verbal Scale* (Calman, 1996; see Table 4.1) is a simple description of the likelihood of an event occurring; its major weakness is the lack of agreement on the definition of the verbal descriptive terms used.

The *Paling Perspective Scale* allows non-technical people to put risks into perspective by comparing them to everyday worries, typically by considering the technical scale used in a subject alongside a common familiar unit (Figure 4.2). It can also be used to compare risks from different options. For more information, see www.johnpaling.com/perspective.html (accessed September 2014).

Another logarithmic scale for expressing risk is the *Community Risk Scale* (Calman and Royston, 1997) which describes a risk in terms of the population unit within which an event

Table 4.1 Calman's Verbal Scale for communicating risk (based on Calman and Royston, 1997).

Risk Range	Risk Magnitude	Risk Description
> 1 in 100	>8	High
1 in 100 to 1 in 1000	8–7	Moderate
1 in 1000 to 1 in 10 000	7–6	Low
1 in 10 000 to 1 in 100 000	6–5	Very low
1 in 100 000 to 1 in 1 000 000	5–4	Minimal
1 in 1 000 000 to 1 in 10 000 000	<4	Negligible

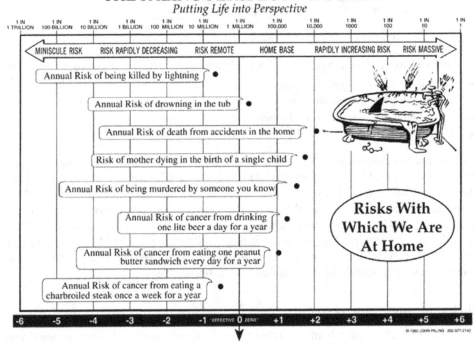

Figure 4.2 Illustration of the Paling Perspective Scale
(source:http://www.johnpaling.com/images/perspectivescalelarge3.jpg

would be expected (see Table 4.2). These authors' goal was to remind health professionals of their obligation to communicate risk in a language with which individuals or groups are comfortable.

Two exercises in risk assessment and communication
What is the risk of vCJD transmission by donor sperm?

In 2006 an attempt was made to answer this question because, even though there was no evidence for any form of CJD ever having being transmitted via human insemination

Table 4.2 Community Risk Scale (based on Calman and Royston, 1997).

Risk	Risk Magnitude	Risk Description*	Example
1 in 1	10	Person	Paying taxes
1 in 10	9	Family	Breast cancer (1:8)
1 in 100	8	Street	Placental abruption
1 in 1000	7	Village	Down syndrome child in women age 30
1 in 10 000	6	Small town	Death by road accident[†],
1 in 100 000	5	Large town	Being murdered[†]
1 in 1 000 000	4	City	Oral contraceptive failure[†]
1 in 10 000 000	3	State or small country	Lightning strike[†]
1 in 100 000 000	2	Large country	Catching measles[†]
1 in 1 000 000 000	1	Continent	Death by space debris (1:5 000 000 000)
1 in 10 000 000 000	0	World	Sexual transmission of vCJD[‡]

* Unit of population in which one adverse event would be expected.
[†] Based on UK statistics c. 1997
[‡] Mortimer and Barratt, 2006

(either coitus or artificial insemination), there were substantial differences in who could be accepted as sperm donors, based on theoretical risks of BSE/vCJD infection (Mortimer and Barratt, 2006). In the USA the FDA regulated sperm donors like blood donors, based on theoretical risks of BSE/vCJD infection: men who had spent more than three months in the UK during 1980–1996, or more than five years in Europe since 1980, were excluded. Yet in Europe and Canada only sperm donor candidates with significant risk factors for CJD were excluded.

Based on survey responses from 18 prion disease experts and 27 sperm cryobanking experts, the risk of a man transmitting vCJD to his spouse was estimated as being <1:10 000 000 in 85% of responses for men in the UK, 91% of responses for men in the rest of Europe, and 98% of responses for men in the USA. On the Calman Verbal Scale <1:1 000 000 is considered a negligible risk (compared, for example to the 1:20 000 risk of a woman dying in childbirth), so 10^{-8} was considered a "trivial" risk.

The study concluded that available data and consensus expert opinion were consistent with a negligible risk of vCJD transmission via donor sperm, and that an ultra-conservative risk avoidance approach would be unlikely to afford increased public safety, while likely reducing treatment options for infertile women. The authors concluded that defining "high vCJD risk" must be based on knowledge rather than fear, and that due caution must be founded upon attempts to quantify real risks rather than avoiding theoretical risks. Why shouldn't infertile women seeking treatment using donor sperm be properly informed of the negligible risk of contracting vCJD, allowed to judge the acceptability of that risk in comparison to everyday risks, and given the choice of accepting sperm from donors screened according to European-style criteria? Unfortunately, it seems that while at least some panel members apparently accepted the study's findings, the FDA was not willing to change its ruling on sperm donors.

The risk of cross-contamination between specimens in cryostorage

A great deal has been written about the risk of possible cross-contamination between samples in cryostorage (review: Mortimer, 2004a). While it is true that the only known occurrence of this involved blood bags (Tedder *et al.*, 1995), and many cryobiologists and embryologists consider it "impossible," the simple fact that numerous government agencies have decided to consider this a real risk (regardless of its possibility being in the "vanishingly small" range) means that it cannot be simply dismissed on either scientific grounds or opinion. Certainly efforts should be made to have regulatory authorities re-evaluate the risk and rank it in real-world terms, but until that happens – and they decide to consider this as reasonable "risk acceptance," IVF labs have no option but to take it into account.

For this reason the current American Association of Tissue Banks (AATB) standards require that "cells and/or tissue shall be processed by methods known to be validated to prevent contamination and cross-contamination," that "reproductive cells and/or tissues shall be stored either in the liquid phase of liquid nitrogen, or provided that the storage method has been validated, in the vapor phase of liquid nitrogen," and that "oocytes and embryos shall be stored in the liquid phase of liquid nitrogen." Yet the vast majority of labs in the USA still package specimens in plastic cryotubes, which have a leakage rate as high as 30% when stored immersed in LN_2...

Similarly, Canadian Standard Z900.2.1–12 *Tissues for Assisted Reproduction* considers this risk in Section 15.6 on "Packaging, Containers and Storage," and concludes that specimens stored in devices that "provide effective biocontainment" are not at risk of causing cross-contamination of other specimens, and are safe from possible cross-contamination if stored in vessels alongside specimens that are known or discovered to be infectious, and shall not be considered as potentially contaminated (Canadian Standards Association, 2012). Basically, this means that if a lab uses devices that have been validated to achieve effective biocontainment (and the only ones that we are aware of at the time of writing are the CBS High Security Straws and Vitrification Devices, see www.cryobiosystem-imv.com) then there is no need for quarantine or isolation tanks, and no need to sanitize tanks.

Process and systems

We have used the terms "process" and "system" several times already in the preceding chapters. To many they are synonymous, but this is not true.

A *process* is defined as a whole series of continuous actions or tasks, or a method by which something is done.

A *system* is defined as a group of objects related or interacting so as to form a unity, or a methodically arranged set of ideas, principles, methods, procedures, etc.

It can therefore be seen that a system is on a more macro scale than a process and, indeed, typically comprises a collection of processes, some of which might occur sequentially, while others might occur simultaneously or in parallel with one or more other processes. At the most basic level, a process can be defined as a single, simple sequence, as illustrated in Figure 5.1.

Systems analysis

A system typically comprises several processes, some of which might run in parallel, but many of which usually operate serially or in sequence, i.e. the output of one is an input to the next.

Systems analysis can be defined as the diagnosis, formulation, and solution of problems that arise from the complex forms of interaction in any system (e.g. from computer hardware to corporations) that exist or are conceived to accomplish one or more specific objectives. The typical use of systems analysis in the IVF Lab is to guide decisions on issues such as planning laboratory operations, resource use and staff/environment protection, research and development, implementing new methods, educational needs, and clinical service provision.

Before a whole system can be understood, there must an understanding of both the individual processes and the environment of extrinsic factors within which each process occurs. The technique whereby a system is best analyzed so it can be understood – or at least represented graphically – is called *process mapping*.

Process mapping

Drawing a process map assists in the development of an understanding of a process, as a first step towards simplifying, improving, or eliminating unnecessary steps (e.g. recursions) in, the process. Process mapping requires that any system or "complex process" be drawn as a flowchart, identifying every step or individual component process in the system. In our case the system of interest is, on the most macro scale, an IVF treatment cycle. But it is essential that the system be reduced to its most fundamental steps for the factors that act upon any (indeed, every) component process to be identified and analyzed. A simple guide to achieving this is to consider each process step as a generic system, one which has inputs

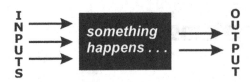

Figure 5.1 A generic process.

to which "something happens" in order to generate the output(s); there must be no lower-level derivative process(es). Unless this level of simplicity is reached the likelihood of success of the analysis will be greatly diminished, if not foredoomed.

A component process will probably have both intrinsic and extrinsic factors affecting its operation:

1. *Intrinsic factors* are those that are inherent to the process, i.e. they are the effects that cause or control the process. The most common intrinsic factors in the IVF laboratory are systems to regulate temperature, pH, and humidity.
2. *Extrinsic factors* are ones that are not inherently involved in the process, e.g. uncontrolled sources of cooling, toxic vapors, biological variation.

In the first edition of this book we considered the preparation of a dinner party as an example of a real-world complex event that included multiple processes, some running in series, others running in parallel. We also referred to the tightly integrated teams that work in major-league restaurants, and likened their functioning to how an IVF Lab operates: each day embryologists must prepare for various procedures, while others are in process, and many of the lab processes must be timed according to their specific biological requirements, and not to the embryologists' – or clinicians' – convenience. By interesting coincidence, 2004 also saw the debut of Gordon Ramsay's *Ramsay's Kitchen Nightmares* TV show, in which he visits restaurants, acts as a troubleshooter, and helps improve the restaurant – all within a week, although with a substantial amount of shouting and cursing.

Since 2000, Oozoa has provided a service to dozens of IVF labs that we call an "operational performance review" or "OPR." After reviewing initial information provided by the subject lab we undertake a three-day site visit, by the end of which we know exactly how the lab does everything in both organizational and technical terms, and we can then provide a report that includes recommendations for improvements. These improvements are designed to improve overall quality, not just in terms of success rates, but also considerations of technical activities, organizational efficiency, ergonomics, and both biological and engineering process optimization, as well as to reduce risk. The philosophy and process of the OPR are entirely based on TQM principles, it does not attempt to consider any specific quality concept such as Kaizen or Six Sigma, nor does it relate to any specific accreditation scheme or ISO norms, although the labs are strongly encouraged to embrace the general principles of ISO 15189. We also achieve this without shouting and cursing!

Extrapolating from these experiences, we have expanded our analogy to consider the more general comparability of operating an IVF center to running a top-flight restaurant. Both employ highly specialized multidisciplinary teams, and there are many similarities in managing the "front of house."

Having considered the integration of processes into complex systems, let's return to the IVF lab and look at how processes make up our operational systems.

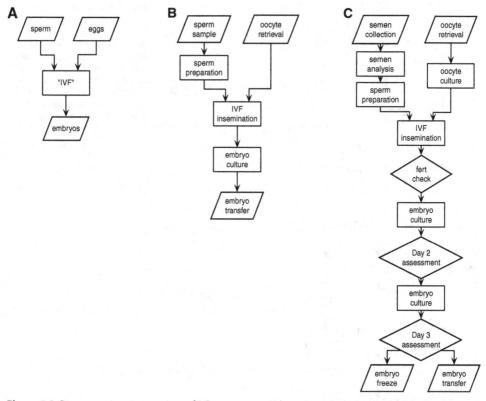

Figure 5.2 Diagrammatic representations of IVF as a process. A shows it at its simplest level, while B and C reveal progressively greater depths of detail in the sequence of generalized stages in the process.

IVF laboratory systems

As we have already said, an IVF treatment cycle is a system, but it is too complex to be analyzed as a single process. To analyze the operation of an IVF laboratory we must "zoom in" on what's going on. Figure 5.2 shows how an IVF cycle can be broken down from a single "black box" process into a series of generalized stages, while Figure 5.3 reveals how the laboratory component of an IVF treatment can be split into a series of procedural steps. Both of these figures illustrate how a more detailed examination of a "system" exposes its lower-order component processes.

However, there are also other dimensions of complexity that arise when one goes beyond a simple IVF treatment cycle to include, for example, the use of previously cryopreserved gametes or embryos (Figure 5.4) or the incorporation of pre-implantation genetic diagnosis (Figure 5.5).

Process mapping tools

We greatly benefited from an excellent primer on process mapping found on the website of John Grout (Grout, 2004); other recommended textbooks include Damelio (1996) and Jacka and Keller (2001). The examples shown in Figures 5.2 through 5.5 were illustrated using the well-known tool of *flow charts*, but there are more sophisticated approaches than

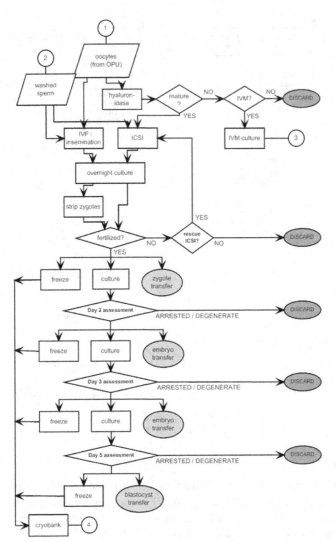

Figure 5.3 A map of the "standard" IVF laboratory process. Off-page connectors relate to: ① the actual oocyte retrieval process; ② obtaining, analyzing, and preparing the sperm sample; ③ the ancillary process of *in vitro* maturation of oocytes; and ④ the process whereby specimens are transferred into the cryobank.

this available to perform process mapping. Some of the more common approaches are listed in Table 5.1, which shows how they differ in their functional attributes. Where temporal analyses are important (i.e. the time taken by processes, e.g. the time to reach certain steps in the process or to complete the process), the more specialized technique called *value stream mapping* can be used, an important tool in the business development process of "lean manufacturing," which was introduced towards the end of Chapter 3.

Flow charts

Flow-charting is the most widely known approach to process mapping and has probably been used by everyone working in IVF labs at some time or another. While flow charts can

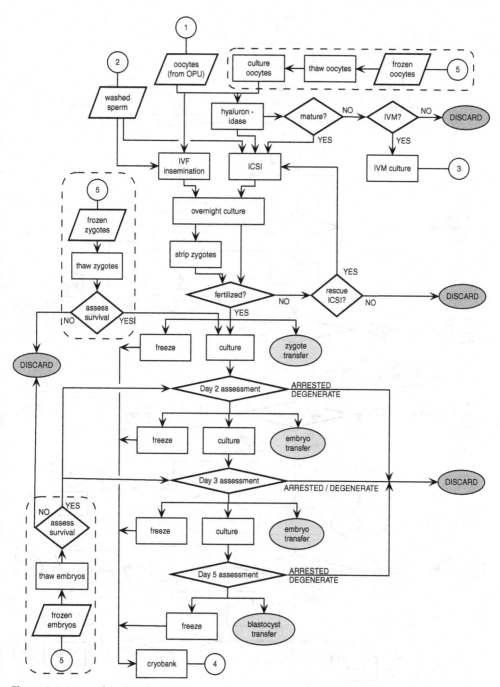

Figure 5.4 A map of the "standard" IVF laboratory process, including the additional complexity of inputs of previously cryopreserved oocytes, zygotes, or embryos. Off-page connectors relate to: ① the actual oocyte retrieval process; ② obtaining, analyzing, and preparing the sperm sample; ③ the ancillary process of *in vitro* maturation of oocytes; ④ the process whereby specimens are transferred into the cryobank; and ⑤ the process whereby cryopreserved specimens are retrieved from the cryobank.

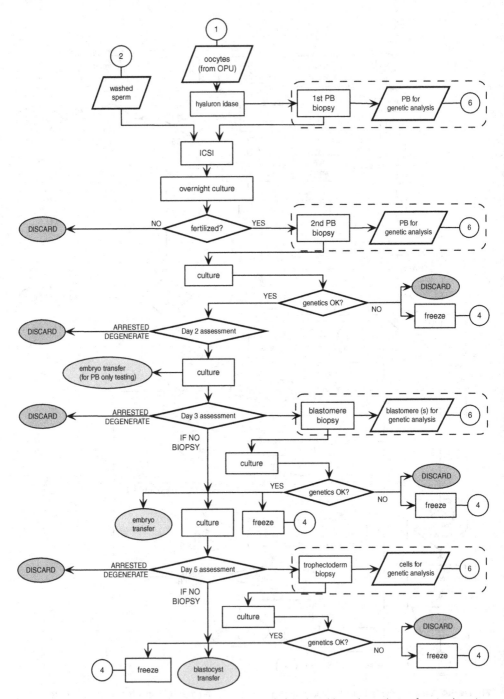

Figure 5.5 A map of the "standard" IVF laboratory process, including the additional complexity of pre-implantation genetic diagnosis/screening. For clarity, rescue ICSI and IVM have been omitted, as well as the inputs of previously cryopreserved oocytes, zygotes, or embryos (see Figures 5.3 and 5.5). Off-page connectors relate to: ① the actual oocyte retrieval process; ② obtaining, analyzing, and preparing the sperm sample; ④ the process whereby specimens are transferred into the cryobank; and ⑥ the processes involved in actually performing the genetic testing on the biopsied material.

Table 5.1 Comparison of the functional attributes of some of the more common approaches to process mapping. "Strong" denotes that the attribute is a strong feature of, or explicit in, the approach; "weak" indicates that the attribute is provided in an implicit or weak way; and a blank denotes that the attribute is not provided by that approach. See text for further discussion of the various approaches. Modified from Grout (2004).

Attribute	Flow charting	Top-down	Swim lanes	IDEF0
Level of detail	Strong		Strong	Strong
Hierarchical linking between maps	Weak	Weak	Weak	Strong
Multiple types of flow	Weak		Weak	Strong
Organizational structure	Weak	Weak	Strong	
Use of icons	Strong		Strong	
Use of logical operators	Strong		Strong	Weak

be accomplished using text only, with various statements inter-connected by arrows, formal flow-charting uses a series of symbols that have specific meanings (see Figure 5.6), although not everyone is aware of these conventions. The amount of detail included in a flow chart is completely at the author's discretion, and large flow charts can be split over multiple pages using the off-page connector symbols. While there is no specific convention in flow-charting to represent any hierarchical structure, greater detail of sub-processes can easily be illustrated using subsidiary "child" flow charts on separate sheets provided that a logical naming or numbering scheme is used to define the linkages (see "IDEF0," below). Multiple flows can obviously be shown in a flow chart, but explanation of what the different flows mean is the author's responsibility.

Various specialized software packages are available for drawing process maps, and flow chart symbols are available in many popular word processing and spreadsheet programs. Probably the most widely acclaimed – and economically priced – flowcharting software package is SmartDraw (SmartDraw.com, San Diego, CA, USA: www.smartdraw.com).

Top-down process maps

These process maps list the main process steps horizontally, with each set of sub-processes listed vertically below the main process steps (Figure 5.7). Because this approach has only very minimal graphical content it is readily usable in text-only situations (Figure 5.8). From this illustration it is obvious that a properly written SOP in a lab manual is, in reality, no more – or less – than a top-down process map.

Swim lane analysis

A swim lane process map is similar to a standard flow chart, except that a grid is superimposed over the flow chart. The analogy is that of swimmers in their lanes in a pool. While the vertical axis or columns of the grid show the chronological sequence of tasks, the grid rows represent the various "participants" (i.e. organizations, departments, functional areas, locations, or individuals) involved in the process. A major strength of swim lane process mapping is that it shows who is involved at each stage in the process; team or joint activities can be indicated by drawing boxes around multiple tasks (Figure 5.9). Because the

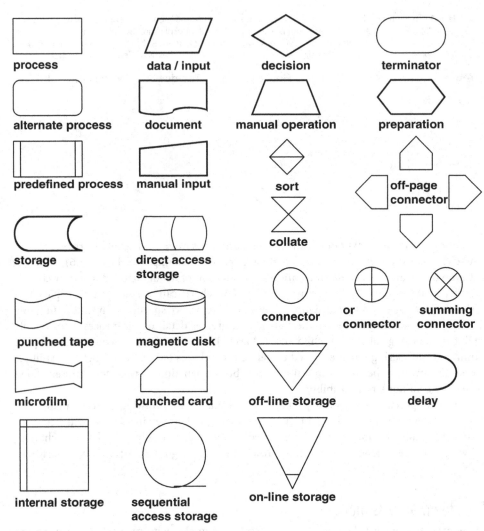

Figure 5.6 Standard symbols used in drawing flow charts.

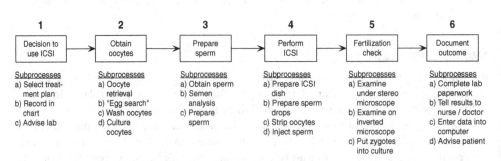

Figure 5.7 The use of ICSI as an example of a top-down process map.

PRE-TREATMENT ARRANGEMENTS

    a) Select treatment plan for patient.
    b) Record decision in patient's medical record.
    c) Advise IVF Lab that ICSI will be used.

LABORATORY PROCEDURES

1. Obtain oocytes.

    a) Oocyte retrieval procedure.
        Details of technical sub-processes go here
    b) Perform "egg search" on follicular aspirates.
        Details of technical sub-processes go here
    c) Wash oocytes.
        Details of technical sub-processes go here
    d) Place oocytes into culture.
        Details of technical sub-processes go here

2. Prepare sperm.

    a) Obtain sperm sample.
        Details of technical sub-processes go here
    b) Analyze sperm sample.
        Details of technical sub-processes go here
    c) Prepare sperm.
        Details of technical sub-processes go here

3. Perform ICSI.

    a) Prepare ICSI dish.
        Details of technical sub-processes go here
    b) Prepare sperm drops.
        Details of technical sub-processes go here
    c) Strip oocytes.
        Details of technical sub-processes go here
    d) Inject sperm.
        Details of technical sub-processes go here

4. Fertilization check.

    a) Examine under stereo microscope.
        Details of technical sub-processes go here
    b) Examine on inverted microscope.
        Details of technical sub-processes go here
    c) Place zygotes into culture.
        Details of technical sub-processes go here

POST-TREATMENT PROCEDURES

    a) Complete lab paperwork.
    b) Advise nurse / doctor of results.
    c) Enter data into the computer.
    d) Advise the patient.

Figure 5.8 An alternate textual view of the top-down process map shown in Figure 5.7. The similarity between this illustration and the format of a laboratory standard operating procedure document is striking.

participants can be defined at a macro or micro scale, on the basis of organizational, functional, or human participants, e.g. roles or actual people, the process can be mapped at whatever level of detail might be desired. If a swim lane process map is constructed using locations then one can also map a process in "geographic" terms, for purposes such as looking at the way biological material – or people, or paperwork – move around (hopefully through) the clinic or the laboratory.

A great benefit of a swim lane process map is that inter-participant exchanges – events that cause the process flow to change "lanes" – can be explicitly stated, e.g. "hand-offs" between the lab and nursing, or lab and physician. This feature alone makes the swim lane approach very useful in IVF where *mistake-proofing* is such an important issue.

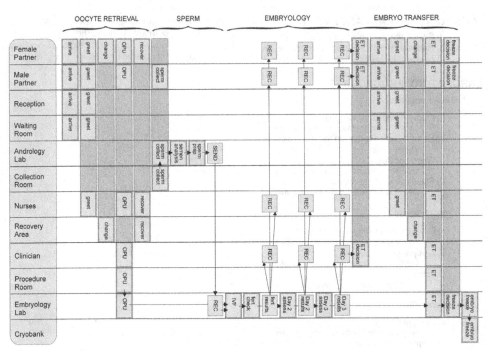

Figure 5.9 The IVF procedure, from oocyte retrieval to embryo transfer, in the form of a swim lane process map that illustrates the movement of the biological material and related information through the organization. Swim lane process maps for a process can be drawn in various ways to emphasize different aspects of the process, entirely according to the user's needs and intentions.

IDEF0

Integration definition (IDEF) is a functional modelling methodology originally developed by the US Air Force to help programmers develop complex software systems. It comprises five separate modelling methods with IDEF0 (pronounced *eye-deff-zero*) being for function modelling. Detailed specifications for IDEF0 were published by the US Government's National Institute of Standards and Technology in 1993 as FIPS publication 183, by which name the source document has since been known (National Institute of Standards and Technology, 1993). Although FIPS PUB 183 is a 128-page document, it is quite (surprisingly?) readable and allows anyone to begin using the technique. The US standard was taken as the IEEE Standard for Function Modelling in 1998, and that Standard (IEEE 1320.1–1998) has officially replaced FIPS PUB 183 as the definitive reference for IDEF0 flow charting (IEEE Standards Association, 1998).

IDEF0 is a totally hierarchical approach to detailed flow chart-based process mapping that uses a completely defined graphical scheme and syntax. While the details of the IDEF0 standard are beyond the scope of this book, the basic element used in IDEF0 flow charts is shown in Figure 5.10. Starting with a single parent map that has only one element, the technique uses multiple, hierarchically linked process maps to display multiple flows in great detail. The IDEF0 specification limits the number of tasks that can be displayed on any single map to being between four and six, and if more steps need to be shown then this is the indication that the process needs to be broken down further and more linked child maps added. Precise numbering of process steps or tasks is at the heart of IDEF0 and allows

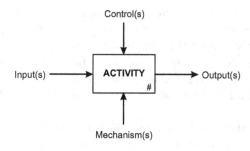

Figure 5.10 A generic illustration of a single element in an IDEF0 process map (National Institute of Standards and Technology, 1993).

ever-increasing detail to be included in the subordinate levels of child maps. An IDEF0 process map is usually accompanied by a table of its levels, known as a "context tree."

At the simplest level, an IDEF0 process map simply shows the details, in a scalable fashion, of the IVF lab processes. As one drills down into the more detailed child maps, the ability to include/show the mechanisms and controls that affect each step of the process (each process "element") comes to the fore, making this probably the most powerful, and most useful, process mapping tool available. An example of an IDEF0 process map is shown in Chapter 7 (Figure 7.6). Certainly both value stream maps and cause and effect (fishbone) diagrams have their roles (see Chapter 3), but the scalability of IDEF0 process maps makes them enormously practical in detailing the complexities of an IVF lab.

Building a process map

Irrespective of the process mapping technique employed, the following outcomes can be anticipated from a successful process mapping exercise:

- Increased understanding of the process;
- Increased consensus among those who created the map about what the process is and how it operates;
- Increased "buy-in" to the need for change; and
- An environment where ideas for process improvement can be generated more rapidly.

When a process mapping exercise is complete, knowledge that has been hidden away inside the heads of many individuals within the organization has been unlocked and is now available throughout the organization. Everyone feels empowered and more confident in their work. Corporate knowledge can be passed on to the next generation without any gaps or misconceptions.

Process mapping usually involves creating a map of the system as it currently operates: the "as-is" map. However, this map should not be created in isolation of the actual process, for example, by the lab director sitting in an office working from the lab manual and other clinic documentation such as the clinical policies and procedures manual, the nursing procedures manual, and the administrative systems manual. The real power of process mapping comes from mapping the process *as it is actually performed, by the people who are actually doing it.* Another concept that we must consider here is whether the process mapping exercise should be performed in a "top down" manner or using the "bottom up" approach. This use of the expression "top down" should not be confused with the specific technique of top-down process mapping.

Here, the "top down" approach is where the lab director, or perhaps a group of managers, draws up the process map, or brings in an external process mapping consultant to do it for them. While this might seem a logical approach, it has several drawbacks:

- As an outsider, the process mapping consultant can only move through the activity logically in a linear manner and, being a non-expert in the technical aspects of the process, the total amount of time required for capturing all the information about the process being mapped is greatly increased.
- By relying on an outsider the IVF center's staff are effectively sidelined and their willingness to "buy-in" fully to the findings and recommendations is consequently diminished.
- The people actually performing the tasks in the process being mapped are denied the opportunity to assess how they, as individuals, are doing their jobs, and hence the chance for them to improve as individuals. A valuable opportunity for self-education is lost.
- Because external consultants are only on-site periodically, the entire process can become fragmented, repeatedly stopping and starting. This makes it difficult to create and build momentum for continuous improvement (see Chapter 3).
- If the organization is pursuing a program of total quality improvement, then there will be many processes requiring mapping, and the continual use of external consultants becomes not only very expensive, but can become the rate-limiting step in the program.

The "bottom up" approach involves staff at all levels directly in the mapping of processes, thereby preventing the adverse effects described for the "top down" approach. It will also allow for faster completion of projects which then encourages their repetition, and in turn fosters the culture of continual change. The end result is therefore a regular series of improvements for the center, rather than a future of continued major effort – and a stream of outside management experts – punctuated by an occasional successful achievement. However, many people working in IVF centers have no experience of process analysis, much less process mapping, and the resultant lack of confidence can be a major hurdle to instituting this essential part of quality and risk management programs. So how should an IVF center go about developing process maps for its activities? Clearly expert assistance is essential, which means that external consultants are extremely useful – if not essential – in the early stages. But they should be brought in as resource people to help staff work through the first few process mapping exercises, and as educators to train staff in performing process mapping so that the organization will be able to undertake a continual series of process mapping exercises using its own staff.

Therefore, a process mapping exercise should proceed as follows:

1. Convene a process mapping team that includes everyone who is involved in the process, or at least a representative of each area or group of workers involved in the process.
2. Have everyone who is involved in the process *independently* review a draft map to identify points of disagreement.
3. The list of points of disagreement is then reviewed by the mapping team to identify errors in the draft map or, more likely, areas where operator-dependent variations have arisen.

Completing the whole mapping process is extremely important because incremental improvements (genuine or otherwise), "coping strategies" or "work-arounds" have often been introduced, frequently without following the proper review and approval procedure,

Table 5.2 Departments or disciplines that can create "silos" that control an organization's operational activities, including explanations of these sources of controlling factors in the generic industrial / commercial and IVF center contexts. Within each of these functional areas the people will generally have a good grasp of that part of the organization's processes and systems to which their work contributes, but often they will not have much knowledge (and less understanding) of what happens in other departments. Achieving understanding of how what they do fits within the company's operations, and how their activities interface with those of other departments is vital to creating a quality organization – the "breaking down of silos."

Department/ discipline	Generic explanation	In the IVF center context
Manufacturing	Where the company's "product" is created.	The actual provision of diagnostic and therapeutic services, including medical, scientific, nursing and counselling activities.
Marketing and sales	Making the company's (potential) customers aware of its products and selling them to those people.	Usually only exists in large "corporate" IVF organizations, but all IVF centers need to be aware of how they get their referrals.
Distribution	Getting the products to the customers.	Not really an issue since the patients come to the clinic. However, in large countries with a low overall population density, e.g. Australia, "outreach" programs have been used very successfully to provide services to patients living outside major metropolitan areas. "Transport IVF" would also come under this area of activity.
Operations	The day-to-day management of the company.	Coordination of the IVF center's activities, including patient appointments, nurse coordinators for treatment cycles, medical records, and scheduling procedures.
Human resources	Recruiting, hiring, training, and supporting the company's personnel.	Of vital importance to creating and maintaining a quality organization – but these activities must be closely integrated into building a multidisciplinary team.
Information technology	Computer systems and software to support all areas of the company's activities.	Just the same functions, although perhaps more important than usual for most commercial businesses in order to achieve efficient management of patients and data handling and analysis for QC/QA, as well as regulatory, purposes.
Finance	Accounts receivable, accounts payable, and financial planning for the company.	Just the same, although perhaps not as well understood as they should be in smaller IVF centers (especially in the public sector).
Legal/ regulatory	Self-explanatory.	Self-explanatory, but perhaps of even greater importance than in many areas of business due to the growing regulation of IVF by government agencies and the expansion of accreditation.

so that often no one person really knows how the entire process is *actually* performed. Anyone who has worked in an IVF lab (or any other lab, for that matter) will know of examples where unauthorized changes ("improvements") were incorporated by individuals, to facilitate their own work, that were not optimal – and sometimes distinctly deleterious – to the overall process. All too often the SOP in the lab manual is not, in fact, the standard operating procedure for a process, a situation that can lead not only to sub-optimal outcomes, but also to increased opportunities for mistakes to occur. Furthermore, process mapping, perhaps especially swim lane mapping, plays a vital role in a comprehensive risk management strategy.

For process improvement, the three steps described above should be followed by:

4. Identify those events in the process map that are the source of either sub-optimal operational performance or outcome, or risk.
5. Create a "to-be" map, showing the team's consensus as to how the process should actually operate after the improvements have been implemented.

Breaking down "silos"

In business management jargon, a "silo" is a single location functional system that is hard to integrate. It might be an operational silo (e.g. the finance department) or a location silo (e.g. a subsidiary facility). Business processes are streams of activity that flow across functional boundaries, e.g. sales, marketing, manufacturing, distribution, operations, finance, legal, etc. (see Table 5.2). Such processes can be described as being fragmented, scattered across so-called functional silos, where people in a given silo rarely, if ever, have occasion or the opportunity to study their work in the context of the larger business process that their function supports. For many people, their company's business processes are literally unknown quantities. It is often said that the only silos that should exist are those for storing grain (since ICBMs are also "user unfriendly"!).

In the IVF world, how many people working at reception, or as nurse coordinators – or even as physicians – actually know what happens in the IVF Lab? The lack of awareness, caused by lack of knowledge, is one of the greatest sources of operational difficulties that the authors encounter when reviewing IVF labs or when a TQM program is being contemplated. In one center where we initiated a program in which all employees working in reception, finance, and nursing were introduced to what went on in the IVF lab, it was such a powerful tool in understanding how the center's systems worked and could be improved, and where "hand-over" errors could occur – essential aspects of preparing for the initial survey for a new accreditation scheme – that this education has subsequently been formalized into the orientation procedure for all new employees. We were so impressed by the success of this pilot scheme that we now recommend it to all our clients.

Process control and process analysis

To analyze a process for either quality management or risk management purposes, one first needs to know the normal parameters of its operation. This requires both reliable information on the historical performance of the process and knowledge of its inherent variability. It is important to think like a statistician – scary as that might seem! Indeed, TQM (of which risk management is one element) requires that scientific method and statistical thought pervade all considerations of process control, performance, improvement, and delivery systems.

The technical aspects of undertaking process control are presented in Chapter 7. However, examples of process control in the IVF laboratory have been described previously (Mortimer *et al.*, 1995; Mortimer, 1999; Murray and Mortimer, 1999) and are slowly being adopted by more and more labs (Wikland and Sjoblom, 2000; Mayer *et al.*, 2003). To decide if a process is sub-optimal, and hence a candidate for improvement, we need knowledge of its capabilities – in other words we need one or more benchmarks for its performance (see Chapter 10).

Identifying controlling factors

Process analysis allows the identification of all the factors that affect the process being analysed. When we write our lab manuals, the SOPs must include sufficient detail for anyone with basic biology lab competence to perform the procedure. The detail must include the precise manner in which the technique is to be carried out. This is especially important in procedures where variations in the technical method can allow either reduced control over factors that can affect the process, or even allow the incursion of extrinsic factors that would otherwise have been excluded. Knowing exactly what must be specified in an SOP to achieve the necessary level of correct technique and standardization, as opposed to being unnecessarily picky, therefore requires that the author of the SOP must understand not just how the process in question is regulated by biology, chemistry and physics, but also how it might be impacted by extrinsic factors or the lab environment, or ergonomics.

Therefore, we are obliged to consider other disciplines such as engineering. Indeed, to identify all the factors that affect how our processes and systems operate in the IVF lab we must consider all of the following:

- Biology
- Biochemistry
- Chemistry
- Physics
- Engineering
- Ergonomics
- Architecture
- Process mapping

Knowing "why", not just "how"

Clearly, writing a good SOP that will include the necessary technical/procedural detail, plus identifying and controlling the other factors that can impinge upon the process, requires far more than just knowing how to do the procedure. Knowing why we do things in certain ways – and also perhaps why we don't do them in other ways – requires more than a simple technical ability to do the task in question. This is why a proper training program for anyone who is to work in an IVF lab must include both the "how" and the "why." Proper training is vital and must be provided within an encompassing framework of education, and the SOPs should constitute the primary source of reference information for trainees about how every aspect of the lab's work is done.

Of course innovations come from people trying different ways of doing things, but the material we handle in an IVF lab is far too precious for empiricism: "suck it and see" has no place in the IVF lab. Learning from history is paramount. If someone has already tried doing something in a particular way and found it to be unsuccessful, or sub-optimal, then there is no value in it being tried again without some other change having been introduced that might alter the course of history the second time around. For example, we know that successful ICSI requires not only that the sperm midpiece must be damaged prior to injection but also that the oolemma must be broken by sucking back on the injection pipette prior to expelling the sperm from the injection pipette. This information came from the many unsuccessful attempts by many of the ICSI pioneers, and these are technical details that every ICSI practitioner was taught at the outset of their training since the earliest days of ICSI's rapid spread outside Brussels. Only someone lacking the necessary knowledge and training, or without any access to the literature (a difficult scenario to imagine if the lab has the resources to buy an ICSI workstation) would perform ICSI without these two "tricks."

Unauthorized variation of methods is a persistent problem in some labs, and is due to either poor training of new scientists or a failure to maintain control over one's staff. Consequently, the problem arises either from a lab director who fails to (re)train new staff, or a failure to recognize – and eradicate – sloppy or lazy behavior by a staff member. And any scientist who will not respect and follow SOPs has no place in an IVF lab.

Tools versus solutions

A common problem when developing new or better processes or systems is confusion between something that is a tool, and something that represents a solution. To illustrate this, let's consider the whole issue of sample identification and verification in the IVF lab, a vital process that extends throughout the entirety of the lab contribution to an IVF treatment cycle.

Obviously each specimen of gametes or embryos must be identified by a label of some description. But because we cannot label the biological material directly we must label the vessel that it is in, e.g. a semen jar, a centrifuge tube, or a culture dish, using perhaps something that is written directly onto the tube or dish, or onto a self-adhesive label that is affixed to the tube or dish (see Figure 5.11). This label needs to identify the source of the biological material inside the tube or dish (its "owner" or "provenance") as well as, most probably, the status of the sample or its stage in the IVF process (e.g. fertilization dish or cleavage dish). The former employs alphanumeric text, and the latter typically either uses the same form of expression or perhaps a color code. But the "label" is only a tool, the reliability of its use depends on the system within which it is used. For example, if the patient's name is Smith (or Jones, Dubois, Patel, Cheng, Ng, etc.) then it is quite likely that specimens from two different people of the same name might be in the lab at the same time. This is why we must use more than just a family name, and why accreditation schemes typically require that any container for a specimen, or preparation made from a specimen, must be labelled with at least two "identifiers" so that the likelihood of ambiguity is eliminated. A family name and first name are obviously inadequate, so a name + date of birth, or name + sample/cycle reference number are needed. The date is clearly not useful for unique identification purposes either, but it is invariably added as further information to facilitate identification of information within the specific patient's record.

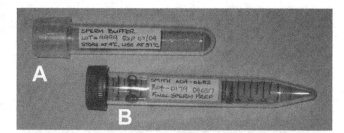
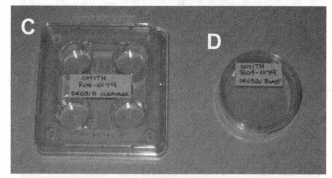
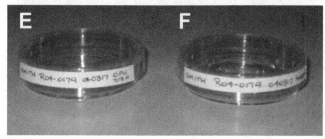

Figure 5.11 Illustrations of the use of labelling in the IVF Lab. Note that each vessel that will contain patient gametes is identified by at least two specific pieces of information, e.g. name and sample/procedure number. Dates are routinely written in YRMODA format to avoid any possible confusion between "/" and the number 1 or the differences between British and American ordering of the date and month. For the aliquot of "sperm buffer" (A) the labelling includes the product name, its lot number, and expiry date, as well as storage and usage conditions, as per accreditation standards. On the label of the sperm preparation tube (B) the reference numbers indicate both the lab reference for the andrology specimen (A04–0682) *and* the oocyte retrieval case number (R04–0179). For the dishes shown as C and D the bottom of the dish must also be labelled, for example either on its edge for C or by backward writing on the base for D. The labels on the dishes shown in E and F are actually attached to the dish bottom but are readable through the side of the lid. All four dishes are labelled with the name, the oocyte retrieval case number, the date, and the purpose of the dish.

With such labelling in place, a sample can be identified unambiguously – and so the only logical conclusion that can be drawn when samples are misidentified is failure of the system within which the label was used. The most common cause of such failures is human error, either misreading hand-written text or actually failing to perform the ID check. The need for diligence and vigilance is compounded by the fact that gametes and embryos must be transferred from one container to another throughout the IVF process. Figure 5.12 illustrates the number of times that the biological materials involved in an IVF treatment are transferred between vessels (at least nine times during a basic IVF treatment cycle), with each change representing an opportunity for error. While everyone working in an IVF lab is aware of the need to perform all these ID verification checks, the system has been known to break down, sometimes with terrible consequences. Occasional errors are made in matching IDs, but the major source of problems here is the failure to verify IDs when the operator is busy. For such reasons, and in response to some events that had very high public profiles, the British HFEA instituted a requirement for a second person to verify the ID check and "witness" the operator performing the process.

But "double witnessing" is a tool, not a solution. Daniel Brison summed up the essence of good laboratory practice very succinctly as "concentration and responsibility" and has

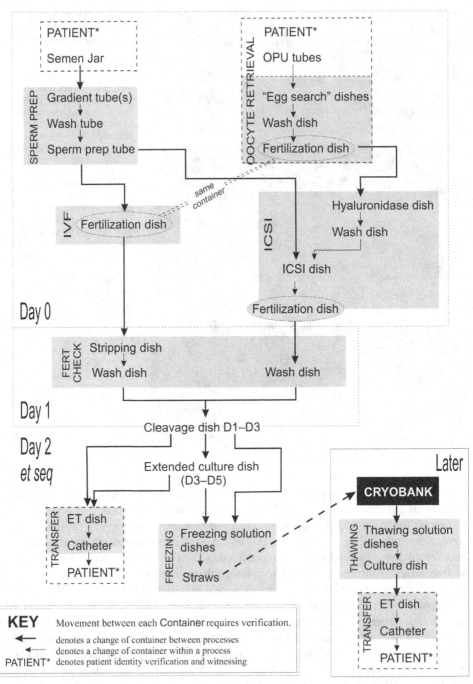

Figure 5.12 A map of the IVF process illustrating all the occasions when gametes or embryos are moved from one container. Each container is defined by a generic name and a change of vessel action is shown by an arrow. *Heavy arrows* show changes of container between general processes and *light arrows* show changes of container between steps within a process. PATIENT* denotes an event where a patient's identity must be verified and witnessed.

presented cogent arguments questioning the efficacy of double witnessing as a safety net for IVF labs and concluded that it has the potential to do more harm than good (Brison *et al.*, 2004). He contends that double witnessing creates two major problems that are in direct conflict with the principles and aims of good laboratory practice ("GLP") and TQM in the IVF lab:

1. The sheer number of times that an embryologist must interrupt their own work to go over and witness someone else's has the effect of destroying the embryologist's concentration on the task-at-hand, increasing the risk that (s)he will make other mistakes not related to specimen identity, thereby compromising the quality of care for the oocytes or embryos. The use of an unskilled dedicated witness probably creates more issues than it solves because the witness needs to comprehend the task being witnessed – as well as the potential sources of error and the possibilities for fraud.

2. Devolving responsibility for the task being performed from the embryologist performing a task (the "primary operator") to the witness of the task can have significant psychological impacts upon those performing laboratory tasks. By requiring double witnessing, the primary operators (regardless of their experience and seniority) are being denied their usual responsibility for accurate specimen handling, much of which now rests with the witness. This perceived loss of responsibility for laboratory paperwork can cause a form of *risk compensation behavior*, a well-known phenomenon in the field of injury prevention, whereby the introduction of preventative measures causes a reduction in the sense of personal responsibility for one's actions or tasks being performed.

While double-witnessing seemed an excellent idea at the time, it must be remembered that "good" IVF labs have, in fact, always focused on specimen identity verification, and that the simple requirement for a second person to sign a lab form does not ensure that positive ID has been verified. Certainly some IVF labs, especially ones that have perhaps a sole embryologist, or where the work hours are protracted due to a high caseload, such a witnessing procedure is not always possible – or is just not always done. Absolute enforcement – and documentation – of such ID checks requires an objective and obligatory technological solution such as Research Instruments' *Witness*, or the *Matcher* or *Trusty* systems (see Chapter 9).

Over the past decade, substantial efforts have been made to use bar codes (Figure 5.13A–D) or RFIDs (radio frequency identification devices; see Figure 5.13E–G) as "more fool-proof" forms of identification for samples. But both RFIDs and bar codes are simply tools, not solutions. Human beings cannot read RFIDs or bar codes – which requires that they be used in conjunction with some "reader" device. While the reader device might be more-or-less infallible in its reading of the RFID or bar code, the actual act of scanning the bar code must be performed – which is open to the same risk of failure as someone not reading any other sort of label. The incorporation of reader devices into workstations so that dishes or tubes cannot be handled without their being read is designed to address this, e.g. as with the *Witness* system (Thornhill *et al.*, 2013).

RFIDs or bar codes can also be transformed from a tool into a process management solution when the need to perform the scan is integrated into some other expanded system, for example, where the bar codes must be scanned in order to enter specimens into a process (e.g. samples being entered into an autoanalyzer machine). Indeed, the first step in implementing *Witness* is to develop a complete process map of your systems,

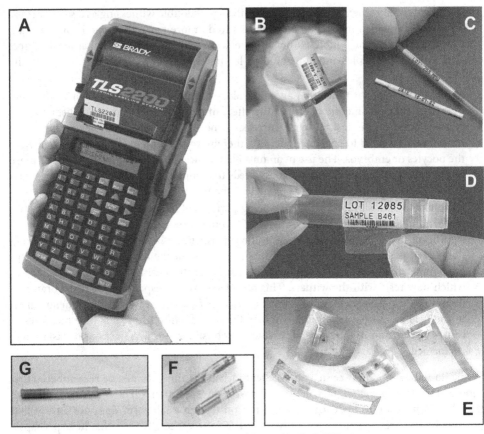

Figure 5.13 Examples of advanced labelling tools: (A–D) bar codes; (E–G) RFIDs.

identifying the critical steps when the biological material is moved from one container or area of custody to another, and using these as check points to ensure the integrity of specimen custody. Figure 5.14 shows the *Witness* process map for the Grace Fertility Centre in Vancouver, Canada, which was the first clinic in Canada to implement this system.

Unfortunately although RFID technology is finding widespread acceptance in identifying vessels containing gametes or embryos during the IVF process, technical problems continue to dog its application in cryobanking – where it would be a great boon for auditing cryostorage tanks. However, a UK company Cryogatt Systems Ltd (see www.cryogatt.com) has recently demonstrated a prototype of such a system.

The importance of these technological advances that allow us to add a machine-readable third identifier to our human-readable label with (at least) two unique identifiers, is rapidly being recognized. Technology such as *Witness* is allowing us to build systems that are less prone to failure – and readily resolve the problem of "lone workers," which many IVF labs suffer at weekends or even during the week in smaller clinics. But it is hard to imagine anyone being willing to rely on an RFID or bar code label as the sole form of identification for a specimen – technology will inevitably be used in conjunction with traditional systems, augmenting human-readable text.

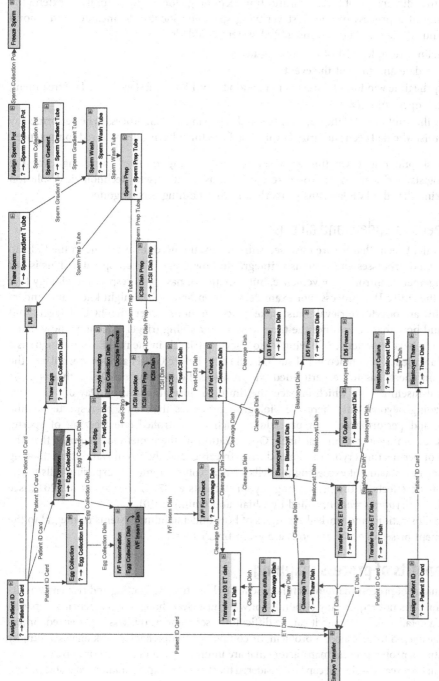

Figure 5.14 An example of a process map for the Research Instruments *Witness* system.

A further dimension of these identification technology tools is their ability to extend the monitoring of a process beyond just verifying specimen identity to include its temporal control and regulation. Such an integrated system could also:

- Maintain a complete list of all pending tasks;
- Log the date and time of the event;
- Verify the time window of the event in relation to the biological stage of the IVF treatment;
- Log the operator's ID;
- Verify the "authority" of the operator (e.g. only allowing an ICSI process to be performed by a scientist who had been authorized by the Lab Director as having the required competence).

While a skeptic might see this as a severe case of "big brother" watching over the embryologists, a risk manager would recognize it as a truly useful technological solution for ensuring that the IVF lab runs properly and that nothing gets forgotten.

Who needs to understand all this?

While it might seem that we are obsessed with details, the need for everyone in the IVF lab to understand processes and systems is integral to how every IVF lab operates. This is not for management control or convenience, but a matter of having to respect the biology that controls the entire IVF process. For example, while embryologists might know and understand why an oocyte retrieval must take place 36 hours after the hCG trigger, and understand how that determines the time window for giving trigger injections, how many are aware or have experience of having to do oocyte retrievals in the middle of the night as a result of a patient's spontaneous LH surge in the days before GnRH agonists? Similarly, the fertilization check has to be performed within a specific window on Day 1 that is 17 ± 1 hours post-insemination, which impacts the timing of inseminations on Day 0.

But going beyond this, there are biological processes that must be respected in the design – and performance – of procedures such as controlled-rate freezing of sperm, embryos, or embryonic stem cell lines. Optimization of these methods requires that the addition of permeating cryoprotectants during freezing, and their removal during thawing must be achieved without exceeding the cells' critical volume limits, or exposing cells to the possible toxic effects of the permeating cryoprotectants at 37 °C (Benson *et al.*, 2012; see also *Fertility Cryopreservation*, edited by Chian and Quinn, 2010).

More illustrations and worked examples of how understanding systems is integral to the development or selection of methods are given in Chapter 11.

The benefits of process mapping

The technique of process mapping is fundamental to both troubleshooting and risk analysis. Its application does not require any elaborate software, just clear thought and a pencil and paper. Without a detailed process map it can be difficult for someone who is less experienced, or less knowledgeable, to troubleshoot a problem, or complete a comprehensive risk analysis. But, by constructing a proper process map, factors that are intuitive to a more expert or knowledgeable person can be revealed – since it can be considered that the more expert or knowledgeable person recognized the factor(s) as important by virtue of having created a mental process map.

This use of *as-is* and *to-be* process maps is integral to the plan, do, check, act, or PDCA, cycle and implicit in performing both a failure mode and effects analysis or a root cause analysis (see Chapter 7).

Making it work

So how do we go about using the principles, techniques, and tools described in the preceding chapters to set up quality management and/or risk management systems in an IVF lab? As we have already said, in truth these goals cannot be limited to the IVF lab, they must involve the entire IVF center, all its operations and all its personnel. However, for the purposes of this book, we can consider some specific areas that are pertinent to the lab that will illustrate how they are inherent to proper lab management.

Methods design and selection

The same principles apply whether we are designing a new (or revised) method ourselves, or selecting one of several variant methods that exist in the literature. When someone in industry wants to have someone make or build something, or perform a task, or provide a service for them, they establish a comprehensive set of criteria specifying all aspects of what is to be done or provided. These specifications are often described as the "user requirement specification" or "URS," and establish the detailed framework within which the work will be done. Creating such specifications is, in reality, a universal principle that can – and should – be applied whenever one individual or organization is supplied a product or service by another.

Particular matters relating to the provision of services by another organization, e.g. estradiol assays by an external endocrine assay lab, are discussed in the following section on "Third-party services." In the present section we will consider the creation of URSs for internal procedures, particularly as they relate to the design or selection of the methods used to perform the component procedures in the IVF process. Consideration of the details of how a procedure (or "task") will be performed is discussed later in this chapter.

There are many facets of a method that must be considered to ensure that the "best" one to meet particular needs is selected. At the simplest level, we need to consider the whole procedure for which we are designing or selecting the method as a process which comprises inputs and actions and generates one or more outputs. Therefore in creating a URS we must include in our analysis the parameters listed in Table 6.1.

It is only after all these parameters have been identified, defined, and understood that you will be in a position to make a sound judgement on the suitability of a method, or whether one technique or protocol is better than another. Then, before implementing the method in your lab, you need to write a comprehensive protocol for the method, covering every aspect, to ensure that the desired outcome will be achieved – and that undesired adverse factors are eliminated as far as technically and/or humanly possible. Writing, and using, lab protocols – or "standard operating procedures" (SOPs), as they are becoming more commonly known – is considered later in this chapter.

Table 6.1 Parameters to be considered when creating a "user requirement specification" or "URS" for a lab method that is to be designed from scratch, modified from an existing technique, or selected from among a number of alternate techniques described in the literature.

Parameter	Comments
Define the overall concept of the method.	Look at the method as a process: define its inputs, actions and outputs.
What is the purpose of the method?	Define the intended purpose of the method as well as those output(s) that can be used as indicators of its performance: e.g. for ICSI the expected proportions of 2PN zygotes that are produced, as well as the rate of oocyte damage during the microinjection procedure.
What is the desired (or required) level of performance of the method?	Establish minimum acceptable levels of performance as well as benchmark levels: e.g. fertilization rate by IVF or ICSI; rapid cleavage rate; proportion of zygotes that reach blastocyst on Day 5.
What are the factors upon which the method is dependent?	These are the factors that control how the method operates, they include technical aspects as well as the underlying biology, chemistry, physics, etc., of the process: e.g. temperature control, pH control, centrifugation force.
What are the necessary characteristics of equipment used to achieve the process?	Define the features of any equipment that will be used to perform the process, including safety, as well as operational performance aspects: e.g. Class II cabinets compared to laminar flow cabinets; the temperature and gas (CO_2) stability of an incubator; the need for swing-out rather than fixed-angle centrifuge rotors – or the need for sealed buckets to avoid aerosol contamination should a tube break during centrifugation.
What are the necessary characteristics of any reagents required for the process?	Define the required features of any reagents, including culture media, that are needed to perform the process, e.g. HEPES versus bicarbonate buffering; minimizing the risk of xenologous contamination.
What are the potential sources of adverse outcome of the method?	These are any factors that can impede the achievement of the intended output(s), including consideration of the quality of the outcome: e.g. failure to control temperature or pH within necessary tolerance ranges.
What are the potential sources of error in the method?	These are primarily the opportunities for human or technical error to impact upon the correct performance of the method and the achievement of the desired outcome (and its quality).
What are the technical requirements for any observations to be made during the method or in determining its outcome?	What instrumentation is required for making the observations, and what are the operational and performance characteristics that are required of that instrumentation: e.g. type of microscope optics or magnification (Hoffman or Nomarski optics versus phase contrast for ICSI).
What is the "uncertainty of measurement" for any	Understand the inherent reliability of observations, counts, etc. Define the required accuracy and precision of

Table 6.1 (*cont.*)

Parameter	Comments
observations that are to be made during the method or in determining its outcome?	observations that are to be made. For example, the numbers of sperm counted in a motility or morphology assessment; or the need for replicate determinations.
What special competence is required for the method?	Identify if any special skills or competence are required to perform one or more of the technical components of the procedure: e.g. expertise in ICSI or embryo biopsy; ... or to perform an observational assessment correctly: e.g. accuracy and precision of sperm concentration, motility, or morphology counts.
Are there any special training or educational requirements necessary for correct performance of the method?	Identify if any special licensing is required to perform one or more of the technical components of the procedure: e.g. needing an ICSI license from the HFEA in the UK.
What quality control procedures are required for correct performance of the method?	Having established the techniques whereby the operational performance or outcome of the method will be established or monitored, how do you ensure that, for example, all your scientists will do it the same? For example: do all your embryologists assess embryo grades according to the same criteria and scales; do all your andrology lab personnel assess sperm morphology in just the same way?

"Third-party" services

Probably the most common service that an IVF lab obtains from another organization or "third party" is estradiol assays for monitoring stimulations. While the supplier – usually a hospital or private pathology lab – will typically be a well-established organization providing a wide range of services to many customers, any accreditation or quality management system will require the establishment of a formal service contract between the IVF lab and the service provider. It is not sufficient for the IVF lab to just assume that, since the pathology provider is such a big organization, they "must be doing things right." The same relationship is true for whoever services the equipment in the IVF lab, whether it be workstations, microscopes, or other equipment, or the company that supplies your culture medium, or the people who remove the biohazard waste, and so on.

A formal service contract describes the exact nature of the relationship between the customer (i.e. you, the IVF lab) and the service or product provider. An example of the points that need to be covered in a service contract with an endocrine assay service is provided in Table 6.2 and the requirements of Section 4.4 of ISO 15189:2012 are summarized in Table 6.3.

A commonly encountered issue with equipment servicing is that service reports often do not include documentary evidence of calibration of the test instrument(s) used to perform the servicing/recalibration, e.g. a copy of the certificate of calibration for each test instrument used. Without evidence that the test instrument was itself properly calibrated there could have been faulty recalibration. We have experienced a situation where a portable CO_2 analyzer was wrongly calibrated during its servicing by a certified biomedical engineering

Table 6.2 Example list of factors that should be considered in a contract with an external endocrine assay service for estradiol levels.

Service aspect	Details
Specimen collection	Location(s) and hours of service Who pays for the phlebotomy supplies Requirement for test requisitions Arrangements for transportation to the testing lab Cut-off time for getting samples to testing lab
Sample identification	Required information
Assay methodology	Method and instrumentation Backup in case of instrument failure Handling out-of-range results
Quality management	Inter- and intra-assay coefficients of variation Satisfactory participation in EQA scheme
Results and reporting	Reporting time: expected/maximum/guarantee(?) Uncertainty of measurement Normal ranges and/or reference values

Table 6.3 Summary of the practical requirements for a medical laboratory to enter into a contract as an external service supplier, based on clause 4.4 of ISO 15189:2012. See the original standard for further details.

Clause	Part	Requirement
4.4.1		• The laboratory must have documented procedures for the establishment and review of agreements for such services. • Each request accepted by the laboratory must be considered an agreement. • Agreements must consider the request, the testing and the report. • The following conditions must be met:
	a)	Adequate definition, documentation and understanding of the requirements of the customers and users, and of the service provider, including the methods to be used (as per clauses 5.4.2 and 5.5 of ISO 15189:2012).
	b)	The capability and resources to meet the requirements of the contract.
	c)	Adequately skilled personnel to perform the testing.
	d)	Appropriate testing procedures that meet the customer's needs (as per clause 5.5.1 of ISO 15189:2012).
	e)	The lab must inform customers and users of deviations from the agreement that impact the results.
	f)	Make reference to any work referred to a referral laboratory or consultant.
4.4.2		Reviews of service agreements must include all aspects of the agreement, and any amendments made after commencement of an agreement must be communicated to all affected parties.

company, causing great problems for the lab director who was trying to establish the correct formulation of pre-mixed gas to achieve the intended medium pH in bench-top incubators in a laboratory located in a mountainous area. See also the MINC faulty calibration issue discussed in Chapter 8.

If no service contract has been agreed then there is no guarantee of the level or quality of service that will be provided. Without such guarantees the IVF lab has no recourse should problems with late delivery of results, or aberrant results, or even unexpected changes in pricing, occur – or be perceived to occur. This is why all IVF accreditation schemes, and quality management systems in general (e.g. ISO 9001) expect to see documentary evidence of the existence of current service agreements or contracts for all services that are supplied to the IVF center by organizations or individuals that are not under its direct control or authority. Gentlemen's agreements, "hand-shake" deals, or arrangements that might have been in place for many years, are not sufficient. In this case, if it's not written down it doesn't exist – and the arrangements have no standing in law.

Standard operating procedures or SOPs

Writing SOPs can be quite a daunting task, especially for a new IVF lab or one that has taken the decision to move from its traditional mode of operation (perhaps as a university-based lab) to a "proper" mode of operation including formal accreditation. There is no absolute standard for what an SOP must contain or look like. However, in the USA the National Council for Clinical Laboratory Standards (NCCLS) has a set of guidelines on how to prepare SOPs (NCCLS, 2002) that are acceptable to accrediting bodies such as the College of American Pathologists (CAP) or the Joint Commission on Accreditation of Healthcare Organizations (JCAHO). For medical laboratories in general, the requirements described in Section 5.5 of the ISO 15189:2012 standard (summarized in Table 6.4) are the "gold standard" for documenting a laboratory procedure or test.

It is the responsibility of the lab director to ensure that the contents of each SOP (or other lab document) are complete, current, and have been properly and comprehensively reviewed. Electronic manuals are acceptable provided that all the required information is included, and they are subject to the same document control requirements as hard copy manuals.

Summary protocols, e.g. as index cards, or any "cheat sheets" prepared by *any member of the lab staff*, are acceptable for use as a quick reference at the workbench, but they too must all comply with all the following requirements:

1. They must correspond to the complete manual;
2. They must be part of the document control system;
3. They must be authorized, and be determined as current, by the laboratory director; and
4. The complete manual must be available for reference.

It is important that no-one has the authority to prepare any abbreviated protocol for any use outside of these requirements, because that would destroy the integrity of the document control system – as well as the lab director's control over laboratory methods.

Technical procedures can be based in whole or in part on instructions for use (e.g. package insert) written by the manufacturer, provided that these instructions: (a) conform to the provisions of clauses 5.5.1 and 5.5.2 of ISO 15189:2012; (b) describe the procedure as it is performed in the laboratory; and (c) are written in the language commonly understood by the staff of the laboratory. Any deviations from such manufacturer's instructions must be reviewed and documented, and any additional information that might be required for the staff to perform the procedure must be documented. Each new version of a "kit" that includes major changes in reagents or procedure must be checked for performance and

Table 6.4 Summary of the particular requirements for a standard operating procedure or lab test as defined in ISO 15189:2012 clause 5.5 "Examination processes". See the original standard for further details.

Clause	Part	Requirement
5.5.1	5.5.1.1	• Selected procedures must have been validated for their intended use. • Operators' identities must be recorded. • Performance specifications for a test must relate to its intended use. • Preferred procedures are those specified in: • "instructions for use" of an in-vitro medical device; • established or authoritative textbooks; • peer-reviewed texts or journals; • international consensus standards or guidelines; or • national or regional guidelines. • (See 5.5.1.3 regarding "in-house" methods.)
	5.5.1.2	Validated methods used without modification shall be independently verified by the laboratory prior to their introduction into routine use.
	5.5.1.3	Tests derived from the following sources must be validated by the laboratory: • non-standard methods; • laboratory designed or developed methods ("in-house" methods); • standard methods being used outside their intended scope; or • validated methods that have been modified. If a method is changed then the influences of those changes on it must be documented and, when appropriate, the method revalidated.
	5.5.1.4	Measurement uncertainty must be determined for each measurement procedure that is used to report quantitative results on test samples. This must include defining performance requirements for the measurement uncertainty, as well as regularly reviewing estimates of it.
5.5.2		Biological reference intervals or clinical decision values must be defined, including documenting their basis, and be applicable to the methods used for testing; this information must be communicated to users.
5.5.3		All procedures must be documented and available in a language commonly understood by the laboratory staff, and be available at appropriate locations. Any summary or quick reference format instructions must be controlled documents and correspond to the complete documented procedure (which must be available for reference). In addition to document control identifiers, documentation must include, when applicable to the testing procedure:
	a)	its purpose
	b)	the principle and method
	c)	performance characteristics as per sections 5.5.1.2 and 5.5.1.3 (e.g. precision, accuracy (expressed as measurement uncertainty), detection limit, measuring interval, trueness of measurement, sensitivity, specificity, etc.)
	d)	type of sample
	e)	patient preparation
	f)	type of container to be used (including any additive that might be required)
	g)	required equipment and reagents
	h)	environmental and safety controls
	i)	calibration procedures (metrological traceability)
	j)	detailed description of the procedural steps

Table 6.4 (cont.)

Clause	Part	Requirement
	k)	quality control procedures
	l)	interferences and cross-reactions affecting the procedure
	m)	principle and procedure for calculating results, including measurement uncertainty
	n)	relevant biological reference intervals or clinical decision values
	o)	reportable interval for examination results
	p)	instructions for determining quantitative results when a result is not within the measureable interval
	q)	alert or critical values, where appropriate
	r)	laboratory clinical interpretation
	s)	potential sources of variation
	t)	references

suitability for its intended use by the IVF lab. Any such changes must be dated and authorized as for other lab procedures.

Having a complete set of written SOPs to show the accreditation surveyors is not the purpose of writing them. SOPs are created to be used in the everyday operation of the lab. Their value transcends being a simple method description and includes a wide range of management and educational features. Each properly written SOP will:

- Ensure that the selected method is being performed or used correctly in a technical sense.
- Ensure that potential adverse or deleterious factors are being controlled.
- Provide a framework for the proper quality control of the procedure.
- Detail how the results of the procedure are to be recorded and communicated to everyone who has been deemed by management to have need of them.
- Serve as the primary technical resource for new members of staff during training.
- Serve as the operational and procedural reference for the proper performance of the method, e.g. to avoid unauthorized "improvements."
- Serve as evidence of what was done in case of future dispute or legal action.

As has been explained previously, developing and writing a good SOP requires a sound understanding not just of the technical procedure being performed, but of everything that affects its performance – an understanding that is based on understanding the process. Using, and respecting, SOPs is no less than an obligation of everyone working in the lab – and quality management depends entirely upon this (see Chapter 3). Moreover – and perhaps more importantly in the modern world – effective risk management is also dependent on the absolute use and respect of SOPs (see Chapter 9).

An example of "good" and "poor" versions of an SOP

At its most basic level, an SOP gives sufficient information to ensure that any person with relevant training will be able to perform the task. However, whether the SOP is written to act simply as an *aide memoire* or as a proper resource and training document will determine its relative usefulness and its value in keeping the lab systems under control. To illustrate how different SOPs can be, we have written two versions of an SOP for sperm washing (Figures 6.1 and 6.2). Figure 6.1 shows an SOP that is sufficient to remind a trained scientist of the reagents

Any Fertility Centre: *Laboratory Procedures Manual:* SOP Lab 013 rev.2004a

SPERM PREPARATION
PURESPERM GRADIENTS

PRINCIPLE
Sperm must be separated from seminal plasma quickly and efficiently for use in IVF.

SPECIMEN
Liquefied semen

REAGENTS
Sperm Buffer
Sperm Medium
PureSperm from Nidacon International AB (Göteborg, Sweden).

Preparing Gradients

Upper layer :   40% v/v PureSperm, prepared by mixing 4 ml of stock PureSperm and 6 ml of Sperm Buffer.

Lower layer :   80% v/v PureSperm, prepared by mixing 8 ml of stock PureSperm and 2 ml of Sperm Buffer.

PROCEDURE
1.   Place the upper layers (1.5 ml of 40% v/v PureSperm) into two 15 ml conical tubes. Then, inject the lower layers (1.5 ml of 80% v/v PureSperm) underneath the upper layers. A clear interface should be visible between the two layers.
2.   Layer liquefied semen onto a pair of PureSperm gradients (up to 2 ml of semen per gradient) and centrifuge at 300 *g* for 20 minutes.
3.   Recover the soft pellet from the bottom of each gradient.
4.   Resuspend in *either* Sperm Buffer if processing for IUI or DI, *or* Sperm Medium if processing for IVF or ICSI.
5.   Centrifuge at 500 *g* for 10 minutes.
6.   Aspirate the supernatant and resuspend the pellet in 1 to 3 ml of fresh Sperm Buffer or Sperm Medium.
7.   Assess the concentration and motility of the washed sperm preparation.

REFERENCES
World Health Organization (1999) *WHO Laboratory Manual for the Examination of Human Semen and Sperm-Cervical Mucus Interaction, 4th edition.* Cambridge University Press, Cambridge, 128pp.

Appended documents : PureSperm package insert (in sheet protector).

APPROVED FOR USE		SOP–Lab013–2004a PureSperm gradients		
REVISION	SCIENTIFIC DIRECTOR		SIGNATURE	DATE
2004a				

Figure 6.1 An example of a "poor" SOP for the process of sperm preparation using PureSperm density gradients.

Any Fertility Centre: *Laboratory Procedures Manual*: SOP Lab 013 rev.2004a

SPERM PREPARATION
PURESPERM GRADIENTS

PRINCIPLE

To be potentially functional, ejaculate spermatozoa must be separated from seminal plasma quickly and efficiently. Prolonged exposure to seminal plasma results in marked declines in both sperm motility and vitality and can permanently diminish the fertilizing capacity of human spermatozoa. Therefore, it is essential that spermatozoa for clinical ART procedures must be separated from seminal plasma as soon as possible after ejaculation.

Background

For a detailed review see Mortimer (2000). In general terms, four basic approaches exist for separating spermatozoa from semen: (1) simple dilution and washing; (2) sperm migration; (3) selective washing procedures; and (4) adherence methods for the elimination of debris and dead spermatozoa. However, it has been established that simple dilution and washing can induce severe damage to the spermatozoa as a result of free radicals generated during the centrifugal washing steps. Furthermore, recent evidence has demonstrated conclusively that the population of spermatozoa separated using a density gradient are not only more functional in terms of their fertilizing ability, but also have fewer nicks in their DNA, and hence will contribute better quality chromatin to the embryo. Consequently, the density gradient method of sperm preparation must be used for *all* clinical applications, including ICSI.

The success of sperm preparation methods is often assessed in terms of their yield of motile spermatozoa. Obviously, the fertilizing capacity of a sperm population after processing is another significant factor which might be particularly important when working with compromised sperm populations such as those recovered from post-retrograde ejaculation urine or cryopreserved spermatozoa.

SPECIMEN

See SOP Lab007 *Sperm Collection – Ejaculated Semen* and also the **Notes** listed below.

- Thoroughly mixed liquefied semen is used as soon as possible after the completion of liquefaction. Liquefaction occurs optimally when semen is incubated at 37°C, and takes 10 to 30 minutes.
- Semen must NOT be mixed using a vortex mixer.
- Samples with increased viscosity must NOT be "needled" (i.e. passed through an 18₀ needle to reduce viscosity by shear force).

REAGENTS

Density gradients that will perform optimally with the vast majority of clinical semen samples encountered in clinical ART are two-step discontinuous gradients with usually 1.5 ml layers of 40% (v/v) and 80% (v/v) PureSperm as the upper and lower layers respectively. Gradients must be prepared on the day of use, although the two layers can be prepared in bulk and stored at +4°C for several weeks if prepared under aseptic conditions (they can also be sterilized using 0.22 μm Millipore Millex-GV filters).

Sperm Buffer	This is a Hepes-buffered culture medium which contains 10 mg/ml of human serum albumin to protect the spermatozoa and can be used under an air atmosphere without compromising the pH. (See SOP Lab005 *Culture Media*).
Sperm Medium	This is a bicarbonate-buffered medium used to resuspend washed spermatozoa that are to be incubated under capacitating conditions, e.g. for IVF. It must be used under a CO_2-enriched atmosphere to maintain the correct pH. (See SOP Lab005 *Culture Media*).
PureSperm	Stock PureSperm (100%) is manufactured by Nidacon International AB (Göteborg, Sweden).

Preparing Gradients

Upper layer :	40% v/v PureSperm, prepared by mixing 4 ml of stock PureSperm and 6 ml of Sperm Buffer.
Lower layer :	80% v/v PureSperm, prepared by mixing 8 ml of stock PureSperm and 2 ml of Sperm Buffer.
N.B.	*For efficiency, prepare 15 ml conical Falcon tubes (#2095) with one of the 1.5 ml layers already in them and Falcon 2003 tubes with 3 ml of the other layer (see Method step #1, below). Store these sets at +4°C and place in the 37°C incubator the night before use to allow temperature equilibration. Do not add the second layer until the day of use.*

Figure 6.2 An example of a "good" SOP for the process of sperm preparation using PureSperm density gradients.

Any Fertility Centre: *Laboratory Procedures Manual*; SOP Lab 013 rev.2004a

CALIBRATION

The centrifuge must be calibrated. To convert its "rpm" settings to g use the equation:

$$g = 0.0000112 \times r \times N^2 \text{ where :}$$

g = desired relative centrifugal force
r = radius of the rotor to the bottom of the tube (in cm)
N = rpm

QUALITY CONTROL

No special procedures required.

PROCEDURE

> **ALL slides or tubes prepared from a semen specimen *MUST ALWAYS* be labelled with at least _two unique identifers_**
> (e.g. Lab Reference Number and the patient's name).

N.B. a) Sterile, conical bottom tubes (e.g. Falcon #2095) must *always* be used for centrifuging spermatozoa – in a swing-out rotor – in order to maximize recovery of the spermatozoa.

  b) *Never* change the centrifugation speeds to try and increase the yield, it will only result in recovering either poorer quality sperm or a dirty preparation.

  c) It is highly recommended that gradients always be prepared and run as pairs to maximize yield and guard against problems that might arise as a result of careless handling of the gradients or sampling after centrifugation.

  d) See below for advice on handling atypical specimens.

1. Using a sterile Pasteur pipette place the upper layers (each 1.5 ml of 40% v/v PureSperm) into two 15 ml conical tubes. Then, carefully add the lower layers (each 1.5 ml of 80% v/v PureSperm) underneath the upper layers. A clear interface should be visible between the two layers. See Figure "Before centrifugation" (below).

    Alternatively, the lower layers can be placed in the tubes first and the upper layers added on top of them. This is particularly useful if one has problems achieving a sharp interface between the two layers using the under-layering method.

2. Layer liquefied semen onto a pair of PureSperm gradients (up to 2 ml of semen per gradient) and centrifuge at 300 g for 20 minutes in a swing-out rotor.

3. For each gradient, using a sterile, long-form Pasteur pipette carefully remove the seminal plasma, upper interface, upper (40%) PureSperm layer and the lower interface and discard; leave most of the lower (80%) PureSperm layer in place. Then, using another clean, sterile, long-form Pasteur pipette remove the soft pellet from the bottom of each gradient by direct aspiration (maximum 0.5 ml) from the bottom of the tube beneath the lower (80%) PureSperm layer. See Figure "After centrifugation" (below).

4. Transfer both pellets to a single clean conical tube and resuspend in *either* Sperm Buffer if processing for IUI or DI, *or* Sperm Medium if processing for IVF or ICSI.

5. Centrifuge at 500 g for 10 minutes.

6. Aspirate the supernatant with a sterile Pasteur pipette and resuspend the pellet in 1 to 3 ml of fresh Sperm Buffer or Sperm Medium as appropriate (see step #4). For IVF or in-vivo insemination transfer to a small culture tube (Falcon #2058), for ICSI leave in the large culture tube (Falcon #2057). Then:

    a) For IUI or DI leave the sample at ambient temperature until it is collected by the nurse for insemination; *or*

    b) For IVF, gas the tube with 6% CO_2-in-air, cap it tightly and place it in the dark at room temperature (i.e. in a cupboard in the Embryology Laboratory); *or*

    c) For ICSI, leave the tube loose-capped and place in a 37°C incubator (i.e. Form a A).

7. Assess the concentration and motility of the washed sperm preparation using a Makler chamber (see SOP Lab012). If available, computer-aided sperm analysis (CASA) may be used.

N.B. a) Even though there will be some (perhaps even 10%) immotile or dead spermatozoa in the final preparation, this is <u>not</u> a problem and there is *NO* need to perform *any* further preparation (e.g. swim-up) as it will have no benefit and could compromise sperm function or survival.

  b) On occasions a washed sperm preparation in culture medium might contain a high proportion of hyperactivated cells that, although very vigorous, may present little progression. In such cases the motility report should state the percentages of progressive

Figure 6.2 (*cont.*)

Any Fertility Centre: *Laboratory Procedures Manual*; SOP Lab 013 rev.2004a

NOTES : Handling atypical specimens

1. **"Dirty" specimens :** If a semen sample contains high numbers of other cells, or is heavily contaminated with particulate debris, the "rafts" formed at the interfaces between either the seminal plasma and 40% PureSperm layers or the 40 and 80% PureSperm layers might be too dense and "clog" the gradient, drastically reducing the yield of spermatozoa. There are several simple steps that can be taken pro-actively to avoid this problem if the semen sample is seen to be very "dirty" on initial microscopic examination:

   a) Only process part of the ejaculate; and/or

   b) Load less semen onto each gradient, perhaps dividing the sample over four gradients instead of two; and/or

   c) Use longer columns of PureSperm, e.g. 2 or 3 ml per layer; and/or

   d) When loading the semen onto the gradient, mix it gently with the upper one-fifth of the upper layer; and/or

   e) Prepare a three-step gradient using layers of 40%, 60% and 80% PureSperm (or 30 / 50 / 80%).

      N.B. *Never use a lower layer of 90% (v/v) PureSperm as this will likely reduce the sperm yield.*

2. **Highly viscous samples :** It can be extremely difficult to obtain good yields of motile spermatozoa from highly viscous samples. To reduce the viscosity and so maximize yield, add an equal volume of Sperm Buffer to the semen sample and mix gently using a sterile Pasteur pipette. If the sample does not disperse within 2 minutes of pipetting, incubate at 37°C for 10 minutes and then mix further. Once the sample has been successfully diluted it can be loaded onto the gradients as usual. An alternative technique for men who are known to have consistently high viscosity is to have them collect into chymotrypsin-coated MARQ™ Liquefaction Cups available from Embryotech Laboratories (Wilmington, MA, USA).

3. **Cryopreserved semen :** Because of the high osmolarity of semen cryoprotectants, cryopreserved spermatozoa will swell greatly upon entering the 40% PureSperm layer and hence decrease their specific gravity. This will not only cause them to be too buoyant to pass through the density gradient, but can also cause impaired sperm function or even survival. To avoid this problem, cryopreserved semen must be diluted with a large volume of "isotonic" medium prior to loading onto the gradients:

   a) Remove the straws or cryovials from the liquid nitrogen. To thaw:

      (i) Straws: Place in a 37°C incubator for a 10 minutes.

      (ii) Cryovials: Allow to stand at room temperature for 10 minutes then unscrew the cap slightly before placing in a 37°C incubator for a further 10 minutes.

   b) Wipe the condensation from outside of the straws or cryovials and then wipe their outsides using 7X detergent.

   c) Straws: Cut off the Critoseal-plugged end of the straw, at the position of the air space, using sterile disposable scissors (Rocket Medical, R50000). Placed the open end in a Falcon #2003 tube and cut the upper cotton-plugged end below the lower wadding to allow the contents to expel into the tube.

      Cryovials: Unscrew the cap and transfer the semen to a round bottom Falcon #2001 tube. If the volume of the sample is >1.5 ml then split it between two tubes.

   d) *Slowly* dilute the semen with a 10× volume of Sperm Buffer, adding it drop-wise with constant gentle mixing over a period of at least 10 minutes.

   e) Layer the diluted specimen onto a pair of PureSperm gradients in conical tubes (Falcon 2095). Up to 3 ml of the diluted sample, or 1.5 ml of fresh semen, can be loaded safely onto each gradient. If necessary, split a diluted sample over 2 pairs of gradients to maximize the yield.

      Alternatively, but sub-optimally, if the total volume exceeds 6 ml the diluted semen can be centrifuged at 500 *g* for 5 minutes (this is safe because the cells that generate free radicals during centrifugation do not survive the freezing & thawing process). Remove the supernatant and resuspend the pellet using 1 to 2 ml of Sperm Buffer. Load this sperm suspension onto the gradients as usual.

4. **Poor quality specimens :** An increased yield can be obtained from most samples, but especially low concentration ones, if slightly less dense layers of PureSperm are used, e.g. 72% and 36% dilutions of PureSperm. However, this only achieved by recovering less dense, and hence less good quality, spermatozoa. It should only be used as a last resort.

5. **Retrograde ejaculate urine specimens :** After the retrograde ejaculate urine specimen has been concentrated by centrifugation and resuspended into a small volume of Sperm Buffer it is layered over two or four PureSperm gradients and processed as per a normal semen sample.

Figure 6.2 (cont.)

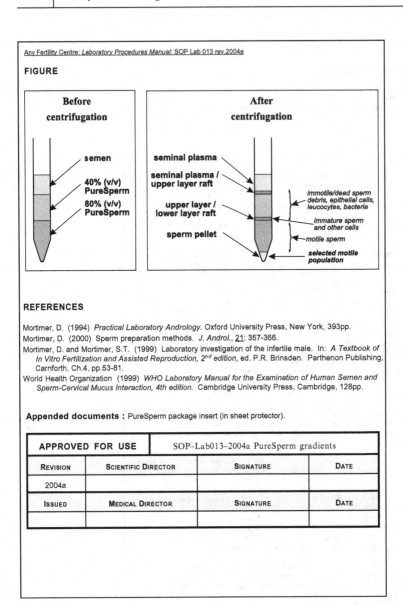

Any Fertility Centre: *Laboratory Procedures Manual*; SOP Lab 013 rev.2004a

FIGURE

| Before centrifugation | After centrifugation |

- semen
- 40% (v/v) PureSperm
- 80% (v/v) PureSperm

- seminal plasma
- seminal plasma / upper layer raft
- upper layer / lower layer raft
- sperm pellet

- *immotile/dead sperm debris, epithelial cells, leucocytes, bacteria*
- *immature sperm and other cells*
- *motile sperm*
- **selected motile population**

REFERENCES

Mortimer, D. (1994) *Practical Laboratory Andrology.* Oxford University Press, New York, 393pp.

Mortimer, D. (2000) Sperm preparation methods. *J. Androl.*, 21: 357-366.

Mortimer, D. and Mortimer, S.T. (1999) Laboratory investigation of the infertile male. In: *A Textbook of In Vitro Fertilization and Assisted Reproduction, 2nd edition*, ed. P.R. Brinsden. Parthenon Publishing, Carnforth, Ch.4, pp.53-81.

World Health Organization (1999) *WHO Laboratory Manual for the Examination of Human Semen and Sperm-Cervical Mucus Interaction, 4th edition.* Cambridge University Press, Cambridge, 128pp.

Appended documents : PureSperm package insert (in sheet protector).

APPROVED FOR USE	SOP–Lab013–2004a PureSperm gradients		
REVISION	SCIENTIFIC DIRECTOR	SIGNATURE	DATE
2004a			
ISSUED	MEDICAL DIRECTOR	SIGNATURE	DATE

Figure 6.2 *(cont.)*

and steps in the procedure. However, it does not offer any background information, or any rules for dealing with atypical specimens. Figure 6.2 is a much more comprehensive SOP, reflecting many years' experience and observation in using this procedure, and illustrating the value of the SOP as a living document. While it gives the same basic information, it includes sufficient background information, procedural details, and rules for dealing with atypical specimens to cover the situations that may be encountered on any given day in an IVF lab. This is important to ensure that all of the laboratory staff members deal with any given situation in a uniform way. This not only helps in troubleshooting, it is also useful when reviewing cycle outcomes, because the procedure used can be removed from the list of potential confounding factors.

The "big nightmare" – did we use the right sperm?

Avoiding this situation is not related to the technical competence of whoever was performing the procedure, but depends on the operator obeying the organizational aspects of a properly controlled process. It has nothing to do with the technical procedure of washing the sperm, or performing the IVF insemination or ICSI, but everything to do with clearing the work area between cases, not processing two cases simultaneously in a way that will create a risk of inadvertent mixing or use of the wrong sperm sample, and of performing the identity checks and verifications that are inherent to the procedure – and which must also be included in the SOP.

Understanding the "hand-offs" or "hand-overs" between stages in a process, or between operators (see the discussion of "swim lane analysis" in Chapter 5 under "Process mapping") – and detailing them in the SOP – is key to ensuring that an SOP contains a complete description of a method that will achieve all its desired outcomes, and avoid known adverse outcomes. "Outcomes" includes organizational aspects of the process, not just its technical endpoint. Therefore, an SOP must include exact descriptions, not just of the series of steps that make up the technical procedure, but also of data recording, results reporting, and, perhaps most importantly of all, the points where operators interact, both within the lab and with other departments, e.g. nursing. Naturally this also then requires verification that each of the other departments' SOPs mirror the described "interface" events.

Managing a cross-departmental process can be facilitated using a checklist type of form that has separate sections for each department (e.g. admin, nursing, lab, medical) with all the steps in the process being shown in chronological sequence, i.e. the order in which they must be performed. If the checklist needs to pass through a department twice, then the sequence of events must be shown this way, e.g. admin → lab → nursing → lab. Constructing this type of checklist form can be achieved very easily using a top-down process map format (Figure 5.8), where each department "visit" is a top level element, and the sequence of steps required within that department are shown as second tier elements under the higher level.

Process control

Again, this is a technique taken from industry, where it was developed to monitor the performance of manufacturing processes. However, rather than compare the performance of a process in relation to some external reference or benchmark, we are monitoring performance relative to the historical performance of our own implementation of a process over time. Basically, by using process control techniques we are able to state whether, at any point in time, our systems are "under control," or not, in comparison with our recent and historical performance levels.

The most frequently used tool is the process control chart or Shewhart chart, named after one of the technique's early proponents, Walter A. Shewhart.

Control charts

Figure 6.3 is an illustrative example of a control chart for a generic process whose outcome is measured using an Indicator that has a range from 0 to 100 (e.g. percentage values). Baseline data on the performance of the process is required for a representative period of operation, e.g. monthly average values for the Indicator over the preceding six months. The

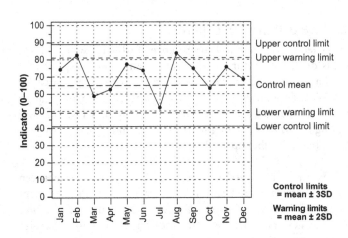

Figure 6.3 A generic control chart (a.k.a. Shewhart chart).

mean and standard deviation (SD) of these six values is calculated and these values used to establish the "control mean" and two types of operational limits: (a) "warning limits," defined as the mean ± 2SD; and (b) "control limits," defined as the mean ± 3SD. The number of prior data periods required to calculate the control limits for an indicator is not pre-determined arbitrarily. The number used must be sufficient to give a good indication of the variability of the indicator, but at the same time not be so many that the standard deviation is reduced to the extent that the control limits become too narrow, with the result that apparent control deviations frequently turn out to be random fluctuations in the indicator. We have used MedCalc software very successfully to produce control charts for many years (MedCalc Software, Mariakerke, Belgium; www.medcalc.be).

It is also true that as a lab becomes better organized, implements more robust methods, or performs more cases per unit time, there will be a reduction in the inherent variability in its Indicators. Under such circumstances the control limits must be re-calculated from more recent data (see below for an example of this).

So long as subsequent periodic mean values remain within the control limits, the process is considered to be "in control." However, there are four principal scenarios that require further action:

1. The Indicator crosses its control limit in the adverse direction. Immediate action is required to determine whether there is a genuine problem and, if verified, to seek its resolution.
2. The Indicator crosses its warning limit in the adverse direction. Action is required to determine whether a problem might exist or be developing.
3. The Indicator shows three consecutive changes in the adverse direction, but does not cross the warning (or control) limit. Action is required to determine whether a problem might be developing.
4. The Indicator crosses its control limit in the beneficial direction. The system should be reviewed to see why it occurred and whether the improvement is sustained (we refer to this as "progress building" – as opposed to troubleshooting). If the improvement is real, then the control limits must be re-defined.

The example shown in Figure 6.4 is based on data for zygote grade (based on a score out of 20) from Mortimer (1999). Monthly average values for the six months preceding the period

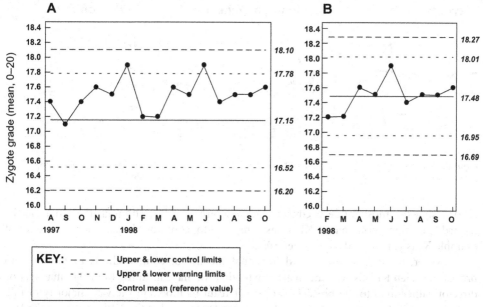

Figure 6.4 A control chart displaying monthly averages for zygote grade (data taken from Mortimer, 1999: see text for explanation). Panel A shows control limits based on the six months preceding the period graphed, while panel B shows re-calculated control limits following the introduction of an improved embryo culture system in mid-August 1997.

shown in Chart A (i.e. February to July, 1997) were used to establish the control mean, and the warning and control limits. However, the introduction of an improved IVF and embryo culture system in mid-August 1997 (see Mortimer *et al.*, 2002a) was the explanation why all the values for subsequent months except one were above the control mean, and this significant change necessitated re-calculation of the control values, using the August 1997 to January 1998 monthly average values, as shown in Chart B. The increased value for the control mean indicates a systematic improvement in zygote grade, while the narrower control limits express the improved stability (i.e. reproducibility) of the new culture system.

A further example, shown in Figure 6.5, illustrates the use of control charts to investigate whether the major re-construction of an IVF lab had any detrimental impact upon the Indicators used to monitor the lab's performance. Since the Indicators during the periods preceding and after the renovations all remained within the previously established control limits, the lab director was able to state with confidence that the renovations had not had any detrimental effect on fertilization rate or embryo quality (Mortimer *et al.*, 2001a).

Previously we have termed the sort of Indicators that are being considered here as "laboratory performance measures" or "LPMs" (Mortimer, 1999; Mortimer *et al.*, 2001a), and in the first edition of this book we harmonized the term as "laboratory performance indicators" or "LPIs." Nowadays, reflecting the more common usage of the ISO expression key performance indicator, all Indicators are now typically referred to as KPIs. Naturally there are other KPIs that can be used to monitor aspects of clinical performance or even of the overall program where the endpoint of interest depends on other sources of variability rather than just the lab methods, conditions, and staff (e.g. pregnancy rate or implantation

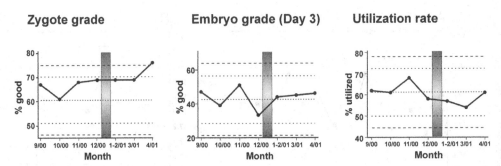

Figure 6.5 A control chart displaying monthly averages for three aspects of laboratory performance before and after a period of major laboratory renovation. Data from Mortimer *et al.* (2001a), see text for explanation.

rate). Using the most modern convention these are all KPIs, although the latter can be termed "program performance KPIs," as compared to laboratory KPIs. An extensive list of example KPIs is provided in Chapter 10.

However, it must be mentioned here that the use of control charts to monitor lab processes via lab KPIs is very much an activity that will have meaning to the lab manager or director rather than to the physicians or other team members in the vast majority of IVF centers. Even if these other team members do understand what the KPIs mean for the IVF center, there is often a perceived "disconnect" between lab operations and pregnancy rates. But when you stop and think about what is actually involved in providing IVF treatment this is not an unexpected – or abnormal – circumstance: after all, the greatest source of variation between treatment cycles is the patients. What KPIs tell us is that the levels of performance of the various lab processes that are being monitored by these Indicators are not straying outside presumably acceptable, historic ranges of variation.

Consequently, monitoring a comprehensive panel of KPIs will allow the lab to provide a rapid response to the seemingly perpetual question of "what's wrong in the lab?" If all the KPIs are within their control limits then the lab can conclusively – and immediately – state that everything is still the same as before, nothing has changed, and hence the questioner should seek an explanation elsewhere for their perceived decrease in whatever endpoint they're looking at. Of course, if a problem does arise then the lab will see it early on – presumably earlier than it will be manifest in any clinical endpoints. The lab will then be able to investigate it and either disregard it as a fluctuation that is not related to any change in operational performance or adverse factor(s) acting on one or more lab processes, or identify the source of the problem and deal with it. In the ideal world it will be the lab that says to everyone else something like "there was a temporary problem with such-and-such, but we've identified the source of the problem and already corrected it."

How "tightly" do we need to control things?

Figure 6.6 illustrates a simplified laboratory in which there are several concomitant processes. However, not all these processes will necessarily have the same periodic (e.g. monthly) variability, or be synchronized, and consequently their net effect over time will be a much higher effective variability in overall performance (e.g. pregnancy rate).

So even if everything is controlled to ±10%, the likelihood that the component processes will be asynchronous means that the overall variability from, say month-to-month, will be

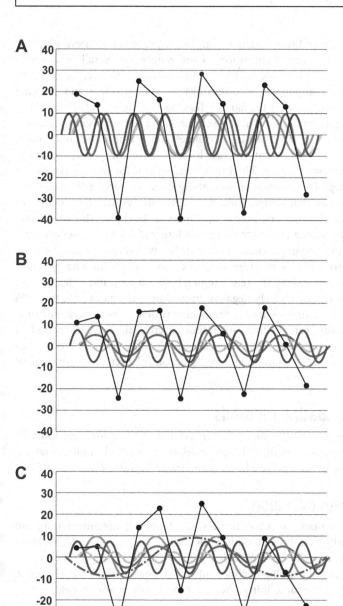

Figure 6.6 Models illustrating how a range of processes, each controlled to ±10%, can interact to affect overall performance. A: Same amplitude (±10%), different wavelengths, generates an effective overall variability ranging from +28% to –39%. B: Different amplitudes (maximum of ±10%), different wavelengths, generates an effective overall variability ranging from +18% to –25%. C: The same general situation as in B, but with an additional, long-wavelength ±10% confounder. In this situation the overall variability is amplified, now ranging from +25% to –31%.

up to three times the amplitude of the individual component processes. Achieving tighter control over at least some of the component processes will reduce the overall variability – but for a clinic to achieve a variation in pregnancy rate of around ±10% (see, for example, Figure 9.7, later) the individual component processes must be well controlled, and reducing that overall variability to ±5% means that the lab is achieving very tight control.

As a corollary to this, Figure 6.6C shows how a serious – and not apparently regular – increase in outcome variability can be caused by a relatively small amplitude confounder, e.g. another component process whose control has broken down, or perhaps is being adversely affected by some extrinsic factor. The importance of this for troubleshooting is obvious: an apparent large negative deviation in something does not necessarily mean that "something big" has happened or gone wrong. Indeed, it is probably yet another example of how a series of small effects can become concatenated, apparently by chance (but in fact due to an alignment of different periodicities), to create a much larger effect that causes concern.

It must be noted that all these examples have modelled the cyclical changes as sine wave fluctuations around the zero effect line. More complex modelling with one or more variables being offset in the adverse direction (e.g. ranging between +3% and –9%), or with an irregular confounder that has an entirely negative impact (e.g. effects of –5% to –15% occurring randomly from time-to-time) will only reveal how widely a macro-scale outcome measure such as pregnancy rate can fluctuate over time, even against a background of relatively small fluctuations in component processes. Clearly the only way that a clinic can achieve stable outcomes is through maintaining very tight control over every component process.

Implementing and validating methods

Practical application of your knowledge about the uncertainty of measurement must be employed throughout the process of method design or selection, method implementation, and method validation. These processes have been summarized in Table 6.5.

Reference materials versus calibrators

These materials are valuable in many aspects of method development, implementation, and validation. They can help verify that the method is being used correctly and in determining its measurement uncertainty, as well as in calibrating instruments, establishing and verifying staff proficiency testing, and in ongoing quality control and quality assurance. However, while many people see them as the same thing, they are not entirely synonymous.

> A *reference material* must be the same as what is being measured, e.g. a panel of serum samples containing known concentrations of a hormone.
>
> A *calibrator*, however, does not need to be the same as what is being measured; it can be a surrogate that is sufficient for certain technical aspects of the method.

A good example here is Accu-beads® (Hamilton Thorne, Beverly, MA, USA). The Accu-bead products are aqueous suspensions of latex particles at known concentrations. In many situations they can be used as surrogates for human spermatozoa, especially when verifying that a counting procedure is being performed correctly. But Accu-beads do not look exactly the same as spermatozoa, and therefore counting them in a specialized counting chamber might well verify the calibration of the counting chamber, but this cannot verify that either the human eye–brain or automated image analysis system recognition

Table 6.5 Sequence of steps in selecting, implementing and validating a method.

Process	Component activity
Method design/ selection	Define what you want to do or measure.
	Review the described/available methods.
	Determine the feasibility of using the method in your lab (equipment, reagents, time, complexity, training).
	Perform a cost analysis.
	Identify the factors that might affect the method's accuracy and precision (uncertainty of measurement).
Method implementation	1. Review all possible sources of error and bias.
	2. Design a method that controls for these problems.
	3. Establish a standard protocol.
	4. Train your staff.
	5. Verify staff performance (proficiency testing).
	6. If necessary, apply corrective action/re-training and
	7. Implement a quality control program for the method.
	8. Participate in an external quality assurance program.
Method validation	Remember: calibration $\neq$ quality control.
	Select appropriate reference materials and calibrators.
	Quality control must be a continual process. Consider process control analysis.
	Participation in an EQAP cannot replace quality control.
	To be useful, an EQAP *must* include both quality assurance and a quality improvement capability.

component of the procedure of identifying and counting spermatozoa would be performed correctly. Accu-beads are excellent calibrators, and have many uses in calibration and quality control, but there are some aspects of the procedures that they cannot verify, and these might require the use of additional materials to ensure full technical competence and proficiency of staff.

Uncertainty of measurement

It is a fundamental principle of the science of mensuration that every measurement has an error associated with it – and that, without a quantitative statement of that error, a measurement lacks worth, even credibility. The parameter that describes, in quantitative terms, the boundaries of measurement error is called the uncertainty of measurement. While "accuracy" is a generally used term and is subject to interpretation, "uncertainty" has a specific meaning, being defined as that parameter, associated with the result of a measurement, that characterizes the dispersion of values that would reasonably be attributed to the measurand (the "measurand" is that particular quantity subject to the measurement). A general background on the uncertainty of measurement can be found in Cook (1999) and the principles governing it are published in the ISO 1993 *Guide to the Expression of Uncertainty in Measurement* – often referred to as the "ISO GUM" (ISO, 1993).

To be meaningful, the uncertainty statement must have an associated confidence level: i.e. the probability that the true value lies within a given range. The most common range

Table 6.6 List of sources of uncertainty in measurement (see ISO, 1993).

Area of uncertainty	Description
What is being measured	Incomplete definition of the measurand. Incomplete realization of the definition of the measurand.
Sampling	Non-representative sampling.
Environmental effects	Inadequate knowledge of the effects of environmental conditions on the measurand (or imperfect measurement of those conditions).
Instrumentation and reading	Observer bias in reading analog instruments or in making subjective assessments. Finite instrument resolution or discrimination threshold.
Standards and reference materials	Inexact values of measurement standards and reference materials.
External factors	Inexact values of constants and other parameters obtained from external sources.
Methodology	Approximations and assumptions incorporated in the measurement method and procedure. Variations in repeated observations of the measurand under apparently identical conditions ("repeatability").

used is the 95% confidence interval (or "95% CI"), which means that there is a 95% probability that the true value lies within the stated range, which is centered around the measurement value. For the mathematically inclined, the 95% CI can be obtained by multiplying the method's combined standard uncertainty of the measurement by 2, although that must have been calculated previously. According to the ISO GUM document, the combined standard uncertainty of a measurement is the square root of the combined variance of the factors creating error in the measurement. However, for the present purpose we only need to understand that no measurement is absolutely accurate, and that we must always endeavor to understand, and be able to provide a good estimate of, the possible dispersion of measured values.

Good laboratory practice requires that all reports express results in particular ways that have meaning and are useful to the intended recipient(s). If this includes a quantitative result, then it should be accompanied by a statement of uncertainty. Determination of that uncertainty typically requires the construction of a model of the measurement system followed by a list of all the factors that can contribute errors to the final result. Clearly this requires a sound knowledge and understanding of the measurement system, as well as the equipment and the environment in which the measurements are made. Yet again, we are confronted with a need to understand process and systems. While detailed considerations of statistical theory and technique are outside the scope of this book, the principles of uncertainty of measurement must be borne in mind when developing or selecting methods, interpreting results or making decisions based on results (see Table 6.6 for a summary of these points, also Björndahl *et al.*, 2010).

Of course, when providing results such as the number of cells in a cleavage stage embryo there is, in most cases, no uncertainty of measurement: the cells present were counted (and, typically, checked), there was no sampling and counting of a hopefully representative

Table 6.7 Relative magnitude of the counting error when basing determinations on small numbers of objects.

Number counted	Counting error
40	±16%
60	±13%
100	±10%
200	±7%
400	±5%

Table 6.8 Limits of the expectation.

Counts	95% confidence interval
4/100	1.74–7.99
5/100	2.43–9.27
6/100	3.15–10.53
7/100	3.89–11.77
8/100	4.73–12.59
9/100	5.51–13.79
10/100	6.6–15

sub-sample. Similarly one might think that measuring the volume of a sample will be "correct," but this is not true: even for a simple aqueous liquid (e.g. culture medium) there will be small errors related to temperature and pipette calibration, as well as perhaps parallax errors when reading the pipette graduations. Obviously the error will be greater when using a less precise device such as a graduated centrifuge tube, and the error can be even larger when working with viscous liquids such as semen. It has long been established that accurate sampling of semen requires the use of a positive displacement pipette, standard air displacement pipettes being subject to substantial inaccuracy when trying to sample a highly viscous fluid. But also we are now measuring ejaculate volume by weight rather than a disposable volumetric pipette (Björndahl et al., 2010), trading off recognizable small errors for potentially much larger errors that the traditional volumetric pipette method is prone to.

Two points of statistical theory are, however, important to note here, especially in relation to such assessments as sperm morphology. These are considerations of sampling error and the reliability of results being related back to a population when they are based on small numbers of observations. Table 6.7 shows the magnitude of simple counting error when making determinations on small numbers of objects counted. Table 6.8 shows the limits of the expectation when a small proportion is determined by counting only a small number of objects, e.g. percentage normal forms based on examining just 100 spermatozoa. Statistics therefore says that a value of 4% normal forms based on a count of 100 sperm might actually be anything from 2 to 8% – and that values of 4% and 7% so-derived are not statistically different.

There are also two main types of error: "random" and "systematic."

Random errors cause lack of precision and arise from chance differences in sampling or reading. These are the errors that we try and minimize by using repeated sampling, or repeated measurements by the same observer, or by the same piece of equipment.

Systematic errors (sometimes referred to as "bias") are far more insidious because they arise from factors that alter the result in only one direction. These shifts in the reported values cannot be detected by repeated measurements.

Minimization of both types of errors is achieved by careful design of the method, analytical instrument selection, adequate sampling and counting, thorough training of the operators, plus internal quality control and external quality assurance components.

All scientists are familiar with results that include references to the standard deviation or the standard error of the mean that establish their place as being representative of a (sample) population. But what about individual results that do not have such qualification? Obviously something like a number of oocytes or embryos is not subject to an uncertainty (beyond the question of whether some might have been missed or lost), but sperm counts or motility assessments can often be very imprecise numbers (see Mortimer *et al.*, 1986, 1989; Mortimer, 1994; World Health Organization, 1999).

How accurate do we need to be?

A final consideration here is "how accurate do the results we quote actually need to be?" There are clearly trade-offs between the costs in time and money of making more accurate quantitative assessments and what the results will be used for. But there is also the obligation that, under the requirements of a quality management system, we must be able to keep the measurement system or assay "under control." If the method has a large uncertainty of measurement then there can be huge fluctuations in results entirely due to technical error and variation, and we have no way of knowing whether a result is genuinely unusual or just comes from the extreme end of the distribution.

Many embryologists (and gynecologists) do not care about the accuracy of sperm counts and related assessments, and will tolerate the use of commonly used, but hopelessly inaccurate, andrology methods on the grounds that the results "make no difference" and/ or "don't help get the patients pregnant." An exhaustive discussion and analysis of the proper management of couples with male factor infertility is clearly not relevant here. However, as scientists we cannot ignore the alternative perception that perhaps had semen analysis results been determined more accurately, it might have been possible to establish them as having greater value in clinical management. There is also some further discussion of this in Chapter 11. As a corollary to this, estradiol values during a controlled ovarian hyperstimulation cycle are only used to establish that estradiol levels are rising comparably to follicular growth – but the assays used must still operate within the standard requirements for accuracy and precision, and expected tolerances of inter- and intra-assay coefficients of variation, in order for the endocrine lab to maintain its accreditation.

A simple answer to the question is, therefore, that any results reported by an IVF lab must be obtained using methods that can be controlled within the constraints of a proper quality management program. As accreditation spreads internationally then more and more IVF labs will have to operate to standards of accuracy and precision for all counts and assessments. Each measurement procedure needs to be validated and its uncertainty established, as per ISO 15189:2012, and as is generally inherent within the EUTCD (see http://ec.europa.eu/health/blood_tissues_organs/key_documents/index_en.htm).

Reference values and ranges

With the publication of the 5th edition of the *WHO Laboratory Manual* ("WHO5") in 2010 there was a flurry of confusion and concern when the reference value for sperm concentration was lowered from 20 M/ml to 15 M/ml, even with the subsequent publication of a large meta-analysis to establish the origin of this new limit (Cooper *et al.*, 2010). In reality, there is a very simple explanation of what this reference limit means: if a man has a sperm concentration <15 M/ml then there is a <5% chance that he fathered a child within the last 12 months. Unfortunately this has minimal clinical value in managing infertility patients since, after all, as he is sitting in the consulting room then, by definition, he did not become a father in the last year... Indeed, what this explanation also reveals is that sperm concentration has very little clinical importance, either diagnostically or prognostically.

Lars Björndahl has published a most erudite discussion of the problems with reference limits in semen analysis and we recommend everyone to read it very carefully (Björndahl, 2011). The basic issue can be summed up by noting that sperm concentration is an indirect expression of whatever pathophysiological problem(s) the man is experiencing that might be responsible for his reduced fertility potential – and since "infertility" is not a simple disease state, such as anaemia or high blood pressure, it is ludicrous to expect the sperm concentration in his ejaculate to be a specific diagnostic criterion. But the problem is far worse than this: sperm concentration in the ejaculate is affected by a whole range of other biological and technical factors that include sexual abstinence, arousal prior to ejaculation, liquefaction of the ejaculate, and technical errors such as incomplete mixing of the liquefied semen, inaccurate sampling and/or dilution, and poor accuracy counting. Based on such understanding comes expectations of minimum standards for semen quality studies (SEMQUA; Sánchez-Pozo *et al.*, 2013).

Clearly it is critical that we understand not just the statistical basis upon which the assumptions of reference ranges and cut-off limits are built, as well as the importance of standardizing analytical methods and practical laboratory training, but also the biological and physiological variability that underlies the characteristics being considered. Only with complete understanding can we expect to be able to make a correct interpretation of not just semen analysis results, but any laboratory result. This issue is discussed further in the ESHRE Andrology SIG's laboratory handbook (Björndahl *et al.*, 2010), which provides far more useful information on interpreting semen analysis values than WHO5 does – if only because it recognizes the need to provide differential interpretation guidelines for semen analysis characteristics depending on whether the endpoint of interest is *in vivo* fertility or *in vitro* fertilization or some other aspect of sperm function.

Equipment specification and validation

Each piece of equipment used in a properly regulated laboratory needs to be selected, installed, validated, and controlled following a standard set of guiding principles.

Design qualification:	The DQ is established by the person responsible for selecting equipment to be used in the laboratory; its purpose is to ensure that the equipment selected will meet the lab's needs, and that it is "fit for purpose."

Installation qualification:	The IQ is performed by a certified engineer (manufacturer or installation contractor) when a piece of equipment or physical plant is first installed to ensure that it is operating in accordance with its design specifications.
Operational qualification:	The OQ is performed by a certified engineer on a regular basis (usually annual, sometimes biannual or biennial) to establish that equipment or physical plant is operating in accordance with its design specifications.
Performance qualification:	The PQ (sometimes called Operational Verification) is performed by a member of staff using appropriate calibrated instruments to verify that equipment or physical plant continues to function within its required operational parameters. It is repeated as often as the user considers is necessary to be confident that the item continues to function as per defined requirements.

Common accreditation requirements for laboratory equipment state:

1. Equipment must be designed and maintained to suit its intended purpose, and must minimize hazards to recipients and/or staff.
2. Critical equipment and devices must:

   A. Be validated, regularly inspected, cleaned, disinfected, and serviced;
   B. Be maintained in accordance with manufacturers' instructions;
   C. Monitor critical parameters: alerts, alarms, and corrective action;
   D. Have measuring functions calibrated against traceable standards; and
   E. Be tested when installed and validated before use [documented].

3. Operational procedures (e.g. SOPs) must include action in case of critical equipment malfunction or failure.

Documenting and maintaining all the records for equipment servicing, calibration, and verification can easily become very arduous, especially if it relies on hard copies. Software options are available for managing many aspects of a QMS, and go far beyond just equipment logging, e.g. Q-Pulse (see www.q-pulse.com).

Document control

An integral part of any quality management or accreditation system is the need for effective document control. A *document control system* will establish and maintain documented procedures for the following requirements:

- Review and approve documents by a competent authority before issue.
- Establish a master document list, and make it available where needed throughout the organization.
- Ensure that all relevant documents are available where and when needed.
- Ensure that obsolete documents are not used accidentally.
- Clearly identify obsolete documents that are retained for any reason (e.g. archived for possible future medico-legal purposes).
- Control the mechanisms for revision of documents.

Table 6.9 Summary of the expectations of ISO 15189:2012 for a document control system. See the original standard for further details.

Clause	Part	Requirement
4.3		A laboratory must control documents that are required by the quality management system, and prevent the unintended use of any obsolete document.
	a)	All documents, including those maintained in a computer system, must be reviewed and approved by authorized personnel before issue.
	b)	Documents are identified by having:a title; • a unique identifier on each page; • the date of the current edition and/or edition number; • pages numbered including the total number of pages (e.g. "Page 1 of 9"); and • authority for issue.
	c)	Current authorized editions and their distribution are identified by means of a list (e.g. document register, log or master index).
	d)	Only currently authorized versions of documents are available at points of use.
	e)	If the laboratory's document control system allows for the amendment of documents by hand pending their re-issue, the procedures and authorities for making any such amendments must be defined. Amendments must be clearly marked, initialled and dated, and a revised document reissued within a specified time period.
	f)	Changes to documents are identified.
	g)	Documents remain legible.
	h)	Documents must be reviewed periodically and updated at a frequency that ensures they remain fit for purpose.
	i)	Obsolete documents are dated and marked as obsolete.
	j)	At least one copy of an obsolete document is retained for a specified time period or in accordance with applicable specified requirements.

Documents subject to an organization's document control system are termed "controlled documents." A more detailed list of the requirements for controlled documents as laid down in Section 4.3 of ISO 15189:2012 has been summarized in Table 6.9. Under this Standard, all documents are considered to comprise part of the organization's quality management system, and a "document" is considered to be "any information or instructions, including policy statements, text books, procedures, specifications, calibration tables, biological reference intervals and their origins, charts, posters, notices, memoranda, software, drawings, plans, and documents of external origin such as regulations, standards or examination procedures."

A copy of each controlled document must be archived for later reference, and this can be achieved using any "appropriate medium" (which might, or might not, include printed hard copy). While it is left to the lab director to define the appropriate retention period, national, regional, and local regulations concerning document retention will often be applicable.

Many accreditation schemes, as well as good practice, require that SOPs be reviewed and reissued annually. They must be signed off by both the laboratory director *and* the medical director. This is important because everything that is done in the IVF lab constitutes part of patient treatment, which must be directed by a clinician. Essentially, the SOPs establish that everything that is done within the lab has been agreed to by the senior physician and so is performed under his/her authority. A corollary of this is, therefore, that so long as the scientists follow the SOPs they ought to be indemnified against any adverse events (see also Chapter 9: "Protecting IVF laboratory staff from unfair litigation"). Even if a problem were to occur as a result of an oversight in a process defined in an SOP, the responsibility ultimately rests with the lead physician who signed off on the SOP, because by signing the SOP they agreed that it would be used in the treatment of their patients. Annual review and reissue ensure that SOPs are current, an aspect that is perhaps even more important in an IVF lab than many other clinical labs due to the rapidly evolving assisted conception field.

However, forms are not "signed off" for use in the way that SOPs are, so we have typically taken a slightly different approach for forms in that they are deemed to remain current unless a new version is created. The identity of the current forms is stated by referencing them in all SOPs in which they are used, and they are therefore effectively reviewed and re-authorized at the same time as the SOPs are re-issued.

Maintaining all the electronic versions of each controlled document requires adherence to strict naming conventions for the electronic files. The following conventions show examples of how we have been doing this over the past couple of decades for several types of documents with a distinction between ones that are re-issued annually (using the year and a single letter qualifier) such as SOPs, and those that remain in effect until changed (using the date they came into effect in YYYYMMDD or "YearMoDa" format) such as forms and job descriptions.

For

SOPs: SOP-Lab001–2014a Short name.EXT

forms: FRM-Lab001-20140317 Short name.EXT

Where:

SOP	denotes that this document is an SOP or protocol
FRM	denotes that this document is a form
Lab	identifies this as a laboratory SOP (rather than a clinical or nursing SOP or protocol)
001	identifies the SOP or form, using a simple sequential numbering system from 1 to 999 (including the leading zeroes makes a list of file names easier to read through).
2014a	denotes the sequence of revisions or issues within the year
20140317	denotes the effective date for the form
Short name	is an abbreviated version of the name of the document to facilitate identifying the correct document when reviewing directory listings in file folders.
EXT	identifies the file type, and hence the software used to create, edit, or print it.

Hyphens are used to separate the various components of the file name for clarity. Other types of document might include:

CON	consent form
EQP	equipment use and care instructions

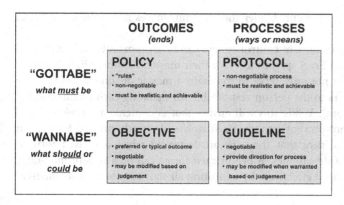

Figure 6.7 Approaches for classifying the purpose of documents.

INF   patient information sheet

INS   instruction sheet

JOB   job description

LST   list

Other documents that should be included in the system are standard or template letters, patient information sheets or handouts, and perhaps also newsletters.

In deciding whether a document is a policy, a protocol, a guideline, or an objective, the principles shown in Figure 6.7 can be useful in resolving uncertainty. Try applying these two approaches to classify the document: does it describe an outcome or a process (i.e. does it relate to an "end" or to "ways" or "means" for achieving that end), or can it be differentiated according to its necessity: a "gottabe" is something that has to be (a "must"), while a "wannabe" is something that should, or could, happen. Of course, a document can also have a composite function, such as has been described in the examples below:

- A policy and a protocol: describing what must be done and the way it must be done.
- A policy and a guideline: describing what must be done and the way that it should or could be done.
- An objective and a protocol: describing what should/could be done and the way it must be done.
- An objective and a guideline: describing what should/could be done and the way it should/could be done.

While implementing and maintaining a document control system takes quite a bit of effort, it does have the very practical benefit of making sure that changes are not accidentally – and hence unpredictably – lost because someone inadvertently uses an outdated document that is somehow still in circulation. As an example, consider how a combined form/checklist might have been updated as an important part of resolving an incident, with the new document having been (re-)designed to ensure that additional safety checks are now part of the routine procedure, with the purpose of avoiding making the same omission error again. But then someone has a stash of already printed copies of the old document, perhaps to save them having to print a copy of the current document each time one is needed, and then fetch it from the printer in the next room. If that person continues to use these copies of the old form the problem could well recur. Under these circumstances how would that affect the clinic's liability?

Maintaining a clinic-wide document control system can be an enormous task, and most clinics do not go beyond using Excel spreadsheets for their master document lists. Software applications are available that not only serve to maintain a master document list but also send out automated reminders to the person responsible for updating each document, e.g. Q-Pulse (see www.q-pulse.com). While this will ensure that documents are reviewed and updated as required, it cannot prevent unauthorized stocks of already printed forms, nor can it help a manager make sure that they are all destroyed when a revised form is introduced. This issue of private supplies of pre-printed forms can be a significant source of risk that can only be managed effectively by educating all staff members of its inherent riskiness.

External quality assurance

Although we have mentioned external quality assurance ("EQA") several times in this book, there are limited options for IVF labs in terms of embryology EQA programs ("EQAPs") at this time. However, one resource that does exist is a web-based commercial service called *FertAid* run by Jim Stanger of Newcastle, Australia (www.fertaid.com) that offers not only EQA but also operates as a training tool and an ongoing educational scheme. FertAid covers both embryology and andrology, and results can be viewed not only in comparison with a peer group, but also within a particular enrolled center, effectively giving it an internal QC dimension as well. However, since the website includes a great deal of material, it certainly needs to be accessed over a good internet connection.

Several andrology EQA schemes exist, and it is extremely important to choose one that includes not only sound quality assurance, but also sound quality improvement functionality. For example, if a scheme only compares your results to those from the other participating labs (even an "all laboratories trimmed mean" or range, where "outliers" have been removed), then it can have no real quality improvement benefit. Similarly, an EQA scheme that provides no suggestion as to the "right answer" must clearly be of limited value. Reference values, even if determined as "consensus" values by averaging the results from a select sub-group of internationally recognized high caliber labs that participate in the scheme, are essential – without them the scheme is "directionless," cannot identify the existence of long-term "drift," and there can be no quality improvement. The ESHRE Andrology Special Interest Group operates an international EQA scheme for semen analysis that is based on a group of reference laboratories, and interested readers should contact Lars Björndahl (e-mail lars.bjorndahl@ki.se) for more information. For more local resources, check with your national andrology society.

Complacency

Although it's a normal human trait, complacency is one of quality improvement's worst enemies. All too often we hear that a lab is "doing alright," or that "we're as good as everyone else" – this is anathema to the philosophy of TQM.

A good example of why we must be vigilant and not succumb to complacency is the situation discussed in Chapter 9, and illustrated in Figure 9.7. This clinic was comfortable with their very respectable overall clinical pregnancy rate of 36.9% per ET, with a month-to-month range of variation of ±10%, results that compared well to other Spanish centers at the time. Following an operational performance review, implementation of the first round of recommended changes led to a highly significant increase in the clinical pregnancy rate of 11.5%, which was accompanied by a halving of the monthly variability in this KPI. The clinic was delighted by the unexpected improvement, and went on to make further beneficial changes.

But what led to the improvements? The first round of changes focused on the basics of ensuring the follicular aspirates were kept warm between the patient and the lab, and that proper physico-chemical conditions were maintained during the examination and handling of oocytes and embryos at the laminar flow cabinet workstations within the embryology lab. The pattern of the change, i.e. a combination of an increased KPI accompanied by a reduction in its variability, is typical of what we have seen many times over the years when embryology lab systems are improved. The long-term benefit was not just a happy client, but a conviction that the principles of TQM work, and ready buy-in from the staff that the changes being proposed would be worthwhile.

Quality and risk management tools

There are many tools available to support quality and risk management in the IVF Lab. However, they are not specific to our field – they are all very well-established generic tools and techniques that have been used for many years in all areas of business.

Inspection and *audit* are observational tools that establish what is happening and whether defined practices are being followed. More in-depth investigations where a process must be analyzed and improved, or risks identified and managed, might need to be undertaken either proactively or retrospectively, for which the most commonly used tools are *failure modes and effects analysis* and *root cause analysis*, respectively.

Finally there is a section illustrating the use of spaghetti diagrams (a common Lean tool) to analyze ergonomics, efficiency, and possible risk aspects of how and where various procedures are performed within the IVF lab. This is another tool that can be applied either proactively, such as during the design of a new laboratory, or retrospectively as part of analyzing an incident or in identifying waste (see Chapter 3).

Inspection

Inspection is simply the careful examination of what goes on in the IVF lab:

- What the environmental conditions are in the lab;
- Whether the lab equipment is working properly;
- What happens in the lab in terms of material and people movement;
- Whether the products used in the lab are appropriate and suitable for use;
- How tasks are performed;
- How information is recorded; and
- How data are analyzed.

It involves the collection, collation, and analysis of data, as well as the examination of processes, which is best accomplished using process mapping. The daily equipment logs maintained by IVF labs following GLP come under this heading, as does the filing of certificates of analysis for each batch of culture medium, and other reagents and routine QC checks on equipment. Unless such information is carefully recorded and/or filed it will not be available if required in a future troubleshooting exercise. People often complain about the amount of paper they have to keep, or that equipment monitoring is "make work" that doesn't help get the patients pregnant. But the certificates of assay and daily log sheets, for example, represent information that could hold the key to solving a problem, perhaps one that *was* stopping the patients from getting pregnant. Meticulous attention to detail and record keeping is vital.

As already mentioned in Chapter 5, we have undertaken operational performance reviews of dozens of IVF labs. At the heart of an OPR is a comprehensive inspection of the lab's systems and processes so that we get to know exactly how the lab does everything in organizational, biological, and technical terms. Only by knowing all these organizational and technical details can we offer recommendations for improvements to increase quality and reduce risk. While this inspection process starts with reviewing SOPs, exhaustive on-site observation of exactly how things are done, combined with discussion of many of the "whys" (and "why nots"), is crucial. Unlike a licensing type of inspection, which seeks only to verify compliance with regulations and can be achieved through the careful application of a checklist, an OPR requires intimate knowledge and understanding of what an IVF lab does, of the underlying biology that pre-determines so much of what needs to be done, and of the ergonomics of practical embryology. In this regard an OPR is a highly specialized inspection or "audit," but something that any well-trained and experienced IVF scientist should be able to undertake, at least of their own systems.

Audit

An audit is a formal examination and verification of an organization's systems or records and supporting documents by a properly qualified professional. It must be an objective activity designed to add value and improve an organization's operations. It helps an organization accomplish its objectives by using a systematic, disciplined approach to evaluate and improve the effectiveness of risk management, control, and governance processes. Audits are undertaken to establish compliance with systems, processes, and SOPs. Any activity in the IVF center can be the subject of an audit, as can the center's success rates.

Guidelines for auditing quality management systems are contained in ISO 19011:2011. Audits must, by definition, be independent and systematic. The basic principles of auditing comprise:

- *Ethical conduct:* As in every activity, ethical conduct, based on integrity, trust, discretion, and confidentiality, is the foundation of professionalism.
- *Fair presentation:* Audit findings, and conclusions drawn, are described accurately and truthfully in the report, along with any obstacles that might have been encountered. Any divergent opinions between the auditors and the organization being audited that cannot be resolved should also be reported.
- *Due professional care:* This reflects the importance of the auditor's task and the confidence placed in them by their clients, other interested parties (e.g. regulatory agencies), and their own employers in the case of professional auditors. It can be summed up as the application of diligence and good judgement.
- *Independence:* In order for audits, and their reports, to be objective and impartial (i.e. free from bias and conflict of interest), auditors must be given independence from the activity or organization being audited.
- *Evidence-based:* An evidence-based approach is the rational method for reaching reliable and reproducible conclusions from a systematic audit. For scientists this obviously reflects the application of scientific method. Although audits only take place within a short time window, it is essential that the information upon which they are based ("evidence") is verifiable and reflects the true nature of the activity or organization being audited.

Our operational performance review is, in effect, a TQM-based audit. To make them less "scary" for the people in the lab that's about to be audited we refer to them as "OPRs" rather than "audits," but they are performed entirely in accordance with the above-mentioned principles. We seek to identify environmental, technical, and operational issues within the ART laboratory that might compromise patient care, fertilization, and embryo development, operational efficiency, or clinical outcomes. We employ a systems analysis approach to evaluate quality management and risk management throughout all the processes that involve the lab and its interfaces with other areas of the clinic, such as medical staff, nursing staff, and administration staff. Upon completion, recommendations are made in a written report (using the usual "must", "should," and "could" qualifiers) of changes that will reduce risk in all its forms, improve quality, improve efficiency, and increase performance (i.e. clinical outcomes). The main conclusions and recommendations are typically presented during an "exit interview" with at least the senior members of the lab team and clinic management, and sometimes – especially in a clinic with a sound quality ethos – even before the entire clinic.

A common confusion when discussing auditing is between what constitutes an *internal audit* and an *external audit*. This differentiation is not so much based on whether the auditor is internal or external to the organization being audited, but the authority to whom they report. When we perform an OPR we are external to the lab being reviewed, but our report is to the clinic's quality committee (or equivalent) for their consideration and decisions on what actions will be taken. We might well refer to matters covered by a professional or authoritative code of practice, ISO standard (e.g. ISO 15189), or regulatory requirement (e.g. as per the EUTCD). However, when a regulatory agency inspector (such as someone from the HFEA) reviews a clinic, (s)he is performing the audit in accordance with the expectations and requirements of the agency, not the clinic – hence this would clearly be an external audit. Another example of an external audit would be a financial audit of a business to confirm its compliance with fiscal regulations.

Failure modes and effects analysis ("FMEA")

Failure modes and effects analysis or "FMEA" is a simple yet powerful engineering quality management technique that helps identify and counter weak points in the design or manufacture of products or the design and execution of processes. Its structured approach (summarized in Figure 7.1) has made it one of the most widely used tools for developing quality designs, systems, and services, and it can be used to improve processes in any organization. Application of FMEA in healthcare typically identifies process components for improvement actions based upon relative ratings of their anticipated frequency and the severity of adverse effects or events.

Conducting an FMEA involves the team following a sequence of generic steps, as summarized in Figure 7.2 and Table 7.1. The first step is to establish the context of the issue and this involves mapping the process so that the details are readily apparent (process mapping has been discussed already in Chapter 5). Possible failure modes can then be identified within the process, each one of which represents a specific risk that is to be considered. The rating schemes for the likelihood and severity of a failure mode or risk are not standardized beyond the organization employing them. In the examples shown in Table 7.2 we have used scales that go up to 10. Even though some organizations employ scales that only go up to five, we believe that the greater dynamic range in assessments that

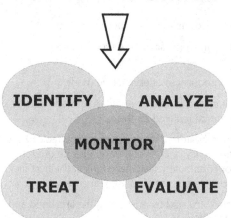

ESTABLISH THE CONTEXT

Figure 7.1 A diagrammatic overview of failure modes and effects analysis (FMEA).

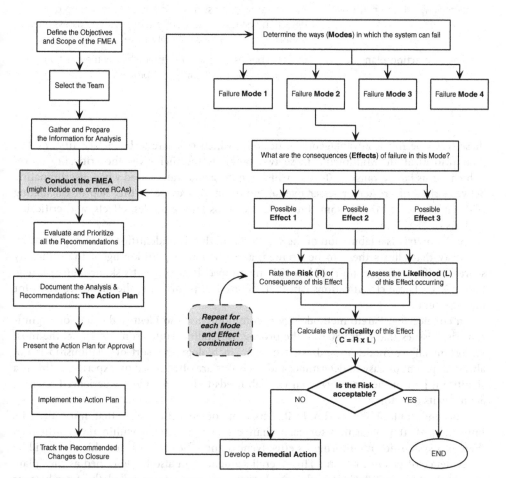

Figure 7.2 A flow chart for performing a failure modes and effects analysis (FMEA).

Table 7.1 The generic steps involved in performing a failure modes and effects analysis (FMEA).

Procedural step	Explanation
Examine and map the process	Identify all the **functions** that are expected to occur.
Identify **failure modes**	Identify any ways in which any of the functions might go wrong.
Determine the **effects**	Establish the consequences of each failure mode.
Identify **contributory factors**	Identify the underlying causes for each failure mode (one or more RCAs might be required for this).
Rate the likelihood and severity of each failure mode	Estimate, using standardized rating schemes (see Tables 7.2 and 7.3), the frequency or likelihood of occurrence of each failure mode or contributory factor, and rank each effect in terms of the possible severity of its consequences.
Calculate the **criticality** of each failure mode (i.e. each risk)	These values are calculated by multiplying the likelihood and severity ranks together.
Identify any existing **controls**	Analyzing the process map, identify any monitoring or detection systems, mitigation systems, etc., and assess their impact on the assigned criticality scores.
Prepare an **action plan**	Identify courses of action and establish how these actions will be assessed for impact upon the process.

these scales permit is advantageous in deciding which risks are to be tackled first, and in their prioritization. Multiplying these two rankings together gives the criticality scores (which for us have a range of 0–100), which are the actual values used when discriminating between risks of greater or lesser overall importance. Because of this step of calculating criticality scores, FMEA is sometimes referred to as failure modes, effects, and criticality analysis or "FMECA."

A *risk matrix* is a tabulation of the scores for all the risks identified by an organization in a way that allows them to be deemed, according to a partitioning of the criticality scores, as (for example) no risk, low risk, medium risk, significant risk, or high risk (e.g. Figure 7.3). These classifications can then be used in prioritizing the identified risks for management.

In engineering, Pareto methodology is commonly used to identify the 20% of "significant risk" issues that cause 80% of the process variability (Hutchison, 1994), i.e. the most important failure modes to address. However, in biology this sort of relationship is not always apparent or easy to determine, and decisions are often based on experience; this is a significant part of the reason why an IVF lab needs to have a senior, experienced scientist acting as its director.

The endpoint of the FMEA is the creation of an action plan that must then be implemented. It is vital that for each change that is instituted within the action plan there is a system for monitoring its effectiveness and efficacy – without this there will be no evidence of positive benefit. This overall sequence can also be described as the "plan, do, check, act" or "PDCA" Cycle (see Figure 7.4), sometimes called the Shewhart or

Table 7.2 A suggested framework for a risk classification scheme comprising risk consequence ("R") and risk likelihood ("L") grading schemes, each on a 0 to 10 scale, for use during risk assessment exercises. Risk criticality ("C") = R × L (range = 0–100), and can be partitioned along the lines of "negligible" (C<20), "low" (C = 20–30), "moderate" (C = 31–48), "high" (C = 49–89), and "extreme" (C ≥90).

Rating	Risk likelihood ("L")	Risk consequence ("R")
0	Impossible – hence it is not a real risk	None – hence it cannot be considered as a real risk
1	Very unlikely: well-controlled or minimized risk, but cannot be completely eliminated	Trivial: in reality there is no measurable adverse risk
2	Unlikely: the circumstances for occurrence are all controlled as far as practically possible, but external factors remain which the organization cannot control	Minimal: in reality the risk is more of a nuisance or inconvenience, with no identifiable impact on patient care
3	Somewhat possible	Quite minor: e.g. impacts the organization's internal systems only
4	Possible	Minor: e.g. definite adverse effect on efficiency but without any measurable effect on treatment outcome
5	Very possible	Quite serious: e.g. definite risk of diminished treatment outcome
6	Quite likely	Serious: e.g. definite adverse effect on patient management or treatment outcome
7	Likely	Very serious: e.g. one or more definite adverse impacts upon multiple patients' management or treatment outcomes, or risk of injury to patients or staff
8	Very likely	Major: e.g. loss of embryos, OHSS, infection of patients or staff, causes actual injury to patient(s) or staff
9	Probable	Extreme: e.g. loss of life, damage to facility (must be at least "very unlikely")
10	Certain: therefore the situation should never exist in the real world	Catastrophic: loss of multiple lives, destruction of facility – in a real-world situation this should apply only to "acts of God," war, or terrorism

Deming cycle (Hutchison, 1994). PDCA-derived knowledge of how a process is currently performing is used to identify and test process changes (improvements). Scientists will immediately recognize the PDCA cycle as a simple expression of fundamental scientific method.

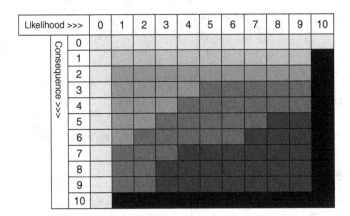

Figure 7.3 An example of a risk matrix.

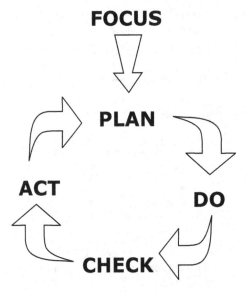

Figure 7.4 The plan, do, check, act or "PDCA" cycle.

Root cause analysis ("RCA")

RCA is a sequence of steps by which the underlying causes ("contributory factors") of adverse outcomes are identified with the goal of preventing the recurrence of such events. Unless an RCA is undertaken with the full support of upper management it might well be performed in a perfunctory manner for the sole purpose of meeting some regulatory requirement.

There is increasing application of RCA in healthcare due to a growing recognition that the complexity of medicine and its delivery is driving the incidence of adverse events (Bogner, 1994; Sharpe and Faden, 1998). Again it must be emphasized that most errors result from faulty systems rather than human error: poorly designed processes put people in situations where errors are more likely occur (Reason, 1994). Risk management experts in all industries emphasize system failures and system-driven errors over direct human error.

The outcome of an RCA will identify three philosophically different types of issues:

1. Blame, responsibility and emphasis on human error;
2. Contributory versus causative factors; and
3. The degree of efficacy of corrective actions or solutions.

To be effective, it must be accepted throughout the organization that RCAs are for improvement purposes and not to assign blame – in keeping with the principles of continuous improvement intrinsic to TQM philosophy.

Because of its history in manufacturing industries, RCA is more readily accepted there by management and employees, compared to healthcare organizations, where it is still typically seen as just another expensive regulatory requirement that does not add value. An additional problem among healthcare workers is a perception that RCAs emphasize human error, raising the specter of blame, litigation, and personal liability. Consequently, there is still resistance to learning about RCAs, resistance to their performance, and lack of support at all levels for their effective application in healthcare.

Undertaking an RCA (see Figure 7.5) is essentially the same as an after-the-fact FMEA and has six stages (see Table 7.3). First and foremost it is essential that everyone involved understands that the goal is to discover everything possible about the incident, with the focus on the systems and processes that could have contributed to the event happening and on the prevention of future recurrence. Every "contributory factor" that has no lower-level derivative is considered to be a root cause. However, when preparing reports one should use the expression "contributory factor" instead of the word "cause"; it is better-received psychologically and has less blatant legal implications.

The goal of an RCA is to develop an action plan that includes at least one corrective action or improvement for each contributory factor that was identified. Before the action plan can be implemented an RCA reporting table is developed, with the following columns for each contributory factor:

- Corrective action(s).
- Person(s) responsible for implementing the corrective action(s). Unless someone is specifically assigned to oversee each corrective action they will not all be pursued, and the expectations of successful outcome will be greatly reduced.
- Action due date. This sets the timetable for each corrective action, which avoids things getting put off indefinitely, as well as giving everyone involved a sense of this being a finite process and a date by which the problem will be resolved.
- Measurement technique. There must be some way of determining that the corrective action has, indeed, had an effect.
- Person(s) responsible for monitoring each corrective action. Again, unless someone is specifically assigned to oversee each corrective action, follow-through can drag on.
- Follow-up date. This is the date by which everyone involved can expect significant progress to have been made.

Depending on the outcome of the RCA, it might be necessary to revise and repeat the RCA process if the problem was not fully resolved.

Using root cause analysis

To illustrate the use of root cause analysis, let us consider an example of troubleshooting where an IVF lab director is concerned about the poor quality of the sperm preparations

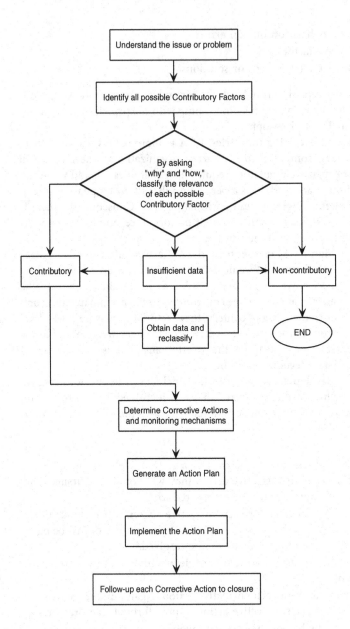

Figure 7.5 A flow chart for performing a root cause analysis (RCA).

that are being produced by the laboratory (see Table 7.4). The pertinent technical background on sperm preparation methods has been extensively reviewed previously (Mortimer, 2000; Mortimer and Mortimer, 1992) and will not be repeated here.

Issue: Even with normal semen samples the sperm preparation method provides a low relative yield (about 15% of the motile spermatozoa initially applied to the gradient) with only 65–70% progressively motile spermatozoa and frequent contamination of the post-gradient sperm population with other cells and debris. A swim-up is

Table 7.3 The six basic stages of performing a root cause analysis (RCA).

Step	Procedure or action	Explanation
1	Understand the issue.	Discover everything possible about the incident, with the focus on the systems and processes that could have contributed to the event happening.
2	Develop a diagram of the contributory factors.	Ask "why?" or "how?" for each contributory factor so that it can be classified as either "insufficient data," "non-contributory," or "contributory."
3	Resolve items classified as "insufficient data."	Obtain data, either by collation, observation, or perhaps even experimentation, for all real or potential contributory factors identified as having "insufficient data," and then re-classifying each of these factors, as appropriate.
4	Generate an action plan.	The action plan should include at least one corrective action or improvement for each contributory factor that was identified. An RCA reporting table is developed for the action plan (see text).
5	Implement the action plan.	Implement both the planned corrective actions and their monitoring processes.
6	Follow-up.	Assess the effectiveness of the corrective actions via the monitoring processes.

needed to improve the motility, but that takes more time and further reduces the yield.

Method: The SOP for sperm preparation in our imaginary IVF lab can be summarized as follows. Apply 1 ml of liquefied semen to a gradient comprised of 0.5 ml layers of 80% and 40% PureSperm (Nidacon International AB, Göteborg, Sweden) in a Falcon 2003 tube. Spin at 2000 rpm for 15 minutes in a Centra CL2 centrifuge fitted with a model 809 rotor. Remove and discard the supernatant (seminal plasma and gradient layers) and re-suspend the pellet in 1 ml of fresh medium. Spin again at 2000 rpm for 15 minutes and again aspirate and discard the supernatant. Repeat the washing cycle. Re-suspend the final sperm pellet in a small volume of fresh medium and overlay with 0.6 ml fresh medium then allow to swim up for 30–60 minutes at 37 °C in a CO_2 incubator. Recover the upper 2/3 of the overlay and assess.

Constructing the RCA: The process map for sperm preparation is shown in Figure 7.6. It clearly illustrates the need to delve deeper until no further subordinate level processes remain because, in reality, the sperm preparation process actually comprises three separate processes. Only by having dissected the process to this level can the following comprehensive troubleshooting exercise be undertaken. The contributory factors and their classifications are listed in Table 7.4. Benchmark criteria are taken from the recommended method for using PureSperm density gradients as per the manufacturer's package insert and previously published information.

Conclusions of the RCA: While the method might not seem to be too different to that used by many other labs, there are numerous factors within the sperm preparation protocol that can contribute to reduced yield in quantitative and/or qualitative terms. In many cases the individual variation might not cause a marked degradation in the outcome, but taken together there will be substantial detrimental impact. The final conclusion is that the sperm preparation method should be replaced by one based on the manufacturer's instructions and established optimized methodology. Furthermore, because this change is not going to have an unknown or uncertain outcome on the process, there is no need to perform any validation studies of the "new" method.

Table 7.4 An example of troubleshooting using RCA to address the issue of "Why do our sperm preparations have variable, and often low, proportions of progressively motile spermatozoa, and are contaminated by other cellular elements and debris from the original semen sample?"

Contributory factor	Classification	Effect	Action	Notes
Gradient colloid concentrations	Non-contributory	Colloid concentrations of 40% and 80% are the recommended layers for PureSperm gradients.	None required.	
Gradient layer volumes	Contributory	Only 0.5 ml layers, this will lead to more rapid "raft" creation and blockage of sperm passage to the lower layer(s) – hence reducing the yield.	Use larger volume layers of 1.5 or 2.0 ml	[1]
Centrifuge tube diameter	Contributory	The tube diameter is relatively small, hence the layer interface area is reduced. This leads to more rapid "raft" creation and blockage of sperm passage to the lower layer(s) – hence reducing the yield.	Use a larger diameter tube, e.g. Falcon 2095.	[1]
Centrifuge tube shape	Contributory	A round bottom tube provides a less discrete pellet than a conical tube.	Use a conical bottom tube, e.g. Falcon 2095.	[1]
Fixed angle centrifuge rotor	Contributory	A fixed-angle rotor means that the pellet will not be deposited in the very bottom of the tube but "smeared" over a larger area of the bottom and one side.	Change to a centrifuge that has a swing-out or swinging bucket type rotor.	[1]

Table 7.4 (cont.)

Contributory factor	Classification	Effect	Action	Notes
Centrifuge buckets are not sealed	Non-contributory	Risk of aerosol contamination in the laboratory if a tube were to break during centrifugation	None in this regard.	2
Centrifugation speed of the first spin	Contributory	The stated rotor has a radius of 12.7 cm, giving a centrifugation force of approximately 570 g which is higher than required.	Decrease the speed to give a centrifugation force of 300 g.	1
Centrifugation time of the first spin	Contributory	Only 15 minutes might not be sufficient for the spermatozoa to reach their isopycnic points on the gradient.	Increase to 20 minutes.	1
Technique for harvesting the pellet from the gradient	Contributory	Removal of all the layers above the pellet exposes the pellet to contamination by residual material from the upper layers that contaminates the inner surface of the tube.	Remove only the seminal plasma layer, the upper (semen/40% colloid) "raft", 40% colloid layer and the 40/80 "raft" to leave most of the 80% colloid layer intact to protect the pellet from contamination. Then harvest the pellet by aspiration through the remaining 80% colloid layer.	1
Re-suspending the pellet in gradient tube	Contributory	The pellet will be contaminated with residual material from the seminal plasma and upper layers (and "rafts" of poor/dead sperm, other cells and debris) that coats the inner surface of the tube.	After recovering the pellet from underneath the remainder of the 80% colloid layer, transfer it to a clean conical tube before re-suspending the cells in fresh culture medium.	1
Centrifugation speed of the second spin	Non-contributory	Although 570 g is is above the recommended 500 g centrifugation force does not become harmful until 800 g.	None required, but the centrifugation speed should be changed to 500 g so as to conform to the standard protocols.	1
Centrifugation time of the second spin	Non-contributory	15 minutes is the usual duration for this spin.	None required.	

Table 7.4 (cont.)

Contributory factor	Classification	Effect	Action	Notes
Harvesting of the washed sperm pellet	Contributory	Because a round bottom tube was used in a fixed-angle rotor the pellet will be "smeared" over a larger area than if a conical tube had been used in a swing-out rotor, rendering complete harvesting more difficult.	Change to a centrifuge that has a swing-out or swinging bucket type rotor and use a conical bottom tube, e.g. Falcon 2095.	[1]
Resuspension of the washed sperm pellet	Non-contributory	None.	None required.	
Performing a second wash step	Contributory	Each wash cycle causes the loss of some spermatozoa, and this could contribute to the perceived low yield.	Since this step is not necessary it should be omitted from the procedure.	[1]
Swim-up from the resuspended washed sperm suspension	Contributory	Although many labs perform such a procedure it is not necessary if the density gradient procedure is performed correctly. The presence of even 15% immotile sperm in the final preparation has never been shown to be harmful to either the fertilization rate or embryo quality.	Do not perform this step.	[1]

Notes:
[1] As per manufacturer's instructions and established optimized methodology.
[2] While this factor is non-contributory to the current issue, it does, however, represent a risk of possible aerosol contamination of the laboratory in case a tube breaks while being centrifuged. In accordance with good laboratory practice the centrifuge should be upgraded to one with sealed buckets. In this case, this could be achieved by only replacing the rotor.

Spaghetti diagrams

These diagrams are created, often on top of a floor plan, to detail the actual physical flow and distances involved in a work process. By enabling a critical analysis of the movement of material or people within the workspace, e.g. the goal of eliminating transit waste, they are well-suited to illustrate a system's inefficiency.

However, a spaghetti diagram can also be used to illustrate an efficient and ergonomic lab design (Figure 7.7); refer to the figure legends for greater explanatory details of the

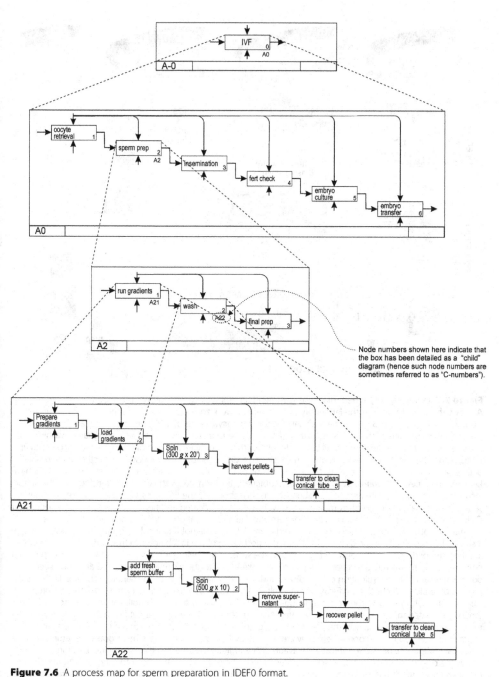

Figure 7.6 A process map for sperm preparation in IDEF0 format.

The first panel shows the obligatory parent process map which is then broken down into sub-processes displayed in multiple, hierarchically linked process maps. Each map should have no more than six steps (although nine could be used without breaking the formal numbering convention). The first map (second panel of figure) shows the basic tasks involved in the process (steps 1 to 6), with step 2 being shown in greater detail in the third panel. The annotation "A2" outside the bottom right-hand corner of step 2 in the six-step chart of process A-0 (its "node number") shows that the box has been detailed as a "child" diagram (i.e. the third panel of the figure). In diagram A2, steps 1 and 2 are identified as being displayed in greater detail in child diagrams A21 and A22 (the fourth and fifth panels of the figure). For clarity, information concerning the controls and mechanisms has been omitted.

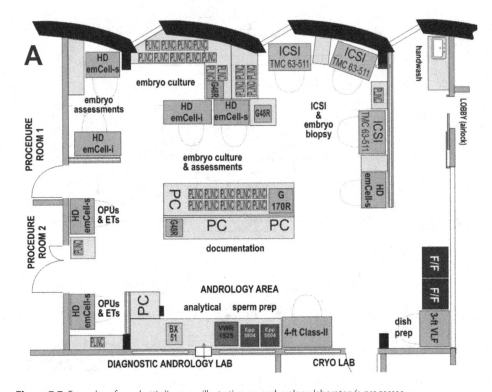

Figure 7.7 Examples of spaghetti diagrams illustrating an embryology laboratory's processes.
A shows the overall layout of the laboratory and its general work zones (see text for further description of the laboratory configuration). **B** shows the material flow for two oocyte retrieval (OPU) procedures "a" and "b" running in parallel, so within each of these processes there are the same four steps: in step 1 the pre-prepared washing and holding dishes are taken from the equilibration incubator to the emCell-s workstation; step 2, which occurs multiple times, is the arrival of the tubes containing the aspirated follicular fluid at the workstation; in step 3 the washed oocytes are transferred from the workstation into the holding incubator (e.g. after a certain number of COCs have been found, or perhaps after each ovary has been aspirated); finally in step 4 the COCs are transferred to the culture incubator in the appropriate area of the laboratory. In this laboratory the IVF cases are handled in an area that is separate from that where the micromanipulation workstations are located and hence where ICSI will be performed. **C** illustrates performing ICSI for a particular micromanipulation workstation: steps 1 and 2 show the movement of spermatozoa and equilibrated hyaluronidase, media, and oil from the holding incubators into the workstation; step 3 shows the movement of the dish of COCs from the post-OPU culture incubator into the workstation. The oocytes are then stripped and the ICSI dish prepared within the workstation before it is taken to the ICSI rig in step 4; after performing the sperm microinjections the ICSI dish is taken back to the workstation in step 5 and the injected oocytes transferred into fertilization culture dishes and then moved, in step 6, to the culture incubator. **D** shows the process of fertilization check for IVF cases being cultured in this area of the laboratory: in step 1 the pre-prepared cleavage dish (and perhaps one or more denudation dishes) is moved from the equilibration incubator into the emCell-s workstation; and the dish(es) of presumptive zygotes are taken from the culture incubator in step 2; after removal of remaining corona cells the presumptive zygotes are transferred at step 3 to the emCell-s workstation that contains an inverted microscope, where they are examined and assessed. In step 4 the zygotes are returned to the emCell-s workstation, transferred into the cleavage dish and finally returned to the culture incubator in step 5. **E** shows the process of embryo assessment for later-stage embryos and their transfer into extended culture: the pre-prepared blastocyst dish is moved from the equilibration incubator into the emCell-s workstation; and the dish(es) of day 3 embryos are taken from the culture incubator in step 2; after evaluation the embryos can be assessed in greater detail on the inverted microscope in the emCell-i workstation (step 3) before being moved back into the emCell-s workstation and transferred into the blastocyst dish and finally returned to the culture incubator in step 4. **F** shows the material flow for two embryo transfer (ET) procedures "a" and "b" running in parallel, so as for OPUs, in each process there are the same four steps: in step 1 the pre-prepared ET dish is transferred from the equilibration incubator to the workstation, and in step 2 the embryos pre-selected for transfer are moved from the culture incubator to the workstation. The ET catheter is the loaded and, in step 3, taken in to the procedure room. If the embryos were not pre-selected then an additional step (4) would involve moving the culture dish containing the remaining embryos back into the culture incubator.

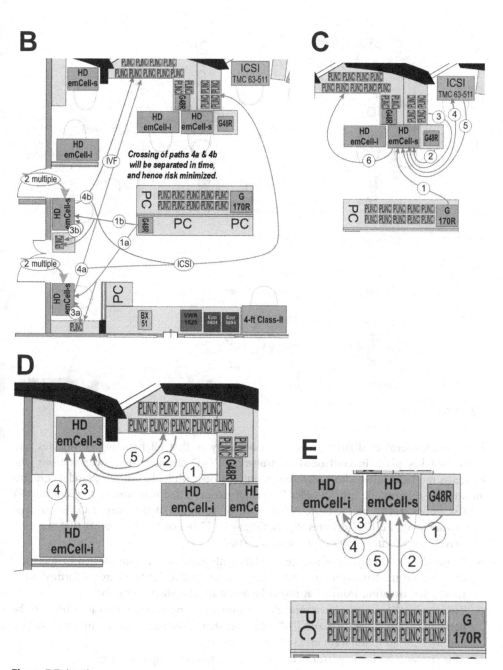

Figure 7.7 (cont.)

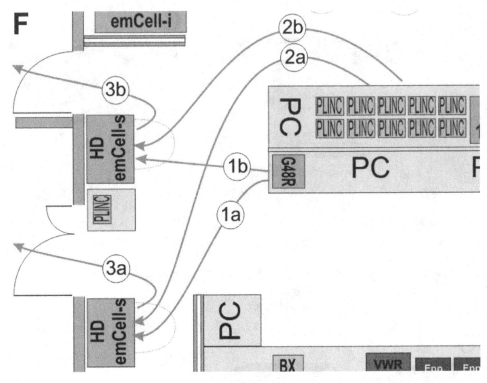

Figure 7.7 (cont.)

processes. General configuration of the laboratory is that all handling of oocytes and embryos takes place in controlled environment "IVF chamber"-type workstations, the emCell-s model is fitted with a stereozoom microscope, while the emCell-i model contains an inverted microscope (e.g. an older ICSI microscope) fitted with modulation contrast or similar optics. G48R and G170R denote Galaxy 48 and 170 liter size, CO_2-in-air type incubators, and "PLINC" denotes Planer/Origio BT37 bench-top incubators that are used exclusively for all culture of oocytes and embryos.

A. Shows the overall layout of a large IVF lab, with various functions located in specific areas within the lab, creating "work zones," where particular tasks are performed with substantial isolation from what might be going on elsewhere in the lab.

B. Two workstations service two procedure rooms, allowing oocyte retrievals (OPUs) to be performed in parallel ("a") and ("b") steps. At step 4, oocytes to be inseminated by IVF and by ICSI go to different areas of the laboratory.

C. This shows ICSI being performed at one of the micromanipulator rigs.

D. IVF fertilization checks, or cleavage-stage embryo assessments, are performed in a dedicated area of the laboratory, using an inverted microscope in the emCell-i workstation for assessing the zygotes.

E. Here later-stage embryos are being assessed, with detailed observations being made on an inverted microscope in the emCell-i workstation.

F. Both procedure rooms can be used for embryo transfers at the same time.

Conclusions

The tools described in this chapter are fundamental to all quality and risk management activities. Familiarity with their principles, and with their use, makes quality and risk management far less daunting prospects. Indeed, with these tools available to you, there is no need to be worried about any of the "scary" concepts or procedures that administrators or business managers, quality managers, and risk managers bandy about, such as "troubleshooting" (see Chapter 8), "risk management" (see Chapter 9), or "benchmarking" (see Chapter 10). As scientists, we already know and understand all the fundamental principles that underpin these tools, and most of them are no more than formalized applications of scientific method.

Once tools like FMEA or RCA have been explained, many scientists exclaim "but that's just common sense!" – and so it is. The real problem lies in the number of people working in IVF (and not just in the lab) who aren't aware of these tools, or can't use them – or, far worse, who don't see the value in their use.

What's gone wrong?: troubleshooting

There are several different conceptual ways of looking at problems (see Table 8.1). While much of this book is about being proactive, no system will be perfect and sometimes you will need to deal with a problem that has occurred or an issue that is affecting the lab, and you will have to be reactive. This chapter is about what to do when things have gone wrong, including dealing with problems and troubleshooting them. Learning how to deal with these subjects is of interest to IVF lab people. Alpha, the international society of scientists in reproductive medicine (www.alphascientists.com), held an internet conference on this subject in 1998 (Elder and Elliott, 1998) and the Alpha workshop at the 11th World IVF Congress held in Sydney in May 1999, was structured as a foundation workshop in reproductive biology that concluded with a session by Jacques Cohen on the practical application of this knowledge in the ART laboratory, with particular reference to troubleshooting.

Having to be reactive

Although we all believe (hope?) that we're doing everything right, that our success rates will be high (and remain high), and that things will continue to run smoothly, we all know that from time to time there will be problems. Sometimes problems are caused by factors outside our control, but sometimes they arise because we have not paid attention to detail, or have not bothered keeping up-to-date on some less interesting aspect of the field, or because someone else (e.g. a supplier) has changed something and either not told us or we did not recognize the importance of the change at the time. Regardless of the origin of the problem, sometimes we have to troubleshoot a part of our system. Of course, the more proactive we are the less likely this event will be, the less serious it is likely to be, and hopefully the easier the problem will be to solve. But sometimes we just have to be reactive. In terms of process analysis, root cause analysis (RCA) is the conceptual basis of troubleshooting.

Troubleshooting

A generic illustration of the troubleshooting process is provided in Figure 8.1. From this flow diagram it is clear that the application of scientific method is fundamental to the process and, indeed, is essential for effective troubleshooting.

Hopefully, many readers will ask "But isn't this all just common sense?" – and the answer would have to be "Yes" – but it is not necessarily so to someone who has not had the benefit of scientific training. For someone who has successfully learned scientific method this structured approach to problem-solving should have become intuitive – and a good scientist will essentially go through all the steps of an RCA automatically, if subconsciously,

Table 8.1 Conceptual approaches to perceiving and dealing with problems.

Action	Nature of problem	Response type	Outcome or effect
Remedial	Existent	Reactive	Alleviate the symptom(s)
Corrective	Existent	Reactive	Prevent recurrence
Prevention	Non-existent	Proactive	Prevent occurrence

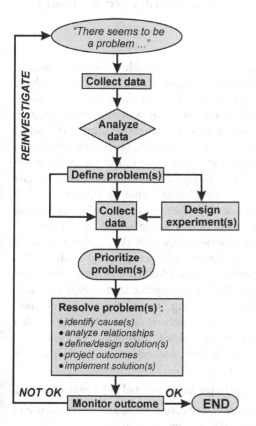

Figure 8.1 An illustration of the troubleshooting process, demonstrating its fundamental equivalence to root cause analysis (RCA). Re-drawn from Mortimer (1999).

whenever they are confronted by a problem. The need to formalize the procedure is to ensure that less-well-trained or less-experienced people can apply the same technique. It also provides the framework whereby the performance of the process is documented – an essential part of all laboratory work, and crucial within the context of accreditation.

An effective troubleshooter can be likened to a scientific detective. Using just the same rigorous objective approach as Sherlock Holmes, one must examine every detail and decide whether it is relevant to the mystery at hand ("contributory" in RCA terminology). Recognizing some of the more obscure factors might require specialist knowledge – from a Dr Watson on your staff – and perhaps failure to recognize such a factor might be a great hindrance to reaching the goal of solving the mystery. This is why it is so important when teaching someone a method that you take the time to explain "why" things are done the way they are (and perhaps why they are *not* done a certain way): just describing the "how" will not produce a truly competent scientist.

Identifying and measuring extrinsic factors that affect a process requires a thorough understanding of the basic science of the process. Not just the biology, but also the chemistry, the physics, and even the engineering that affect the process, as and when required. Without such comprehensive knowledge, your ability to minimize or eliminate the problems will be greatly compromised. In Chapter 13 we have provided an illustrative, but comprehensive, description of how a "well-controlled" IVF lab might be set up, not just in terms of how the systems are intended to operate, but also the control mechanisms that might be put in place to ensure that each process or system continues to function within its expected parameters.

Troubleshooting a biological process

An example of needing to look at many systems together when troubleshooting is illustrated in an investigation of low fertilization rates. It had been shown in numerous studies that a low-glucose environment was beneficial for embryo development from the zygote to the eight-cell stage, and so many laboratories used this type of medium in place of the glucose-containing medium that they had previously used for all of the gamete handling, fertilization, and early embryo-development steps. In some of these laboratories, the fertilization rate by IVF (rather than ICSI) was not as good as hoped, but the cleavage rate of the embryos was very good. A side-effect of this outcome was that some people tended to see IVF as a more "risky" approach than ICSI, in terms of "guaranteeing" fertilization, so there was a shift towards a higher proportion of ICSI than IVF cycles. Whether this was a good or a bad thing is highly debatable – but since it isn't really the focus of this example, we'll leave it there.

The reason for the lower-than expected fertilization rates with IVF, and the relatively higher fertilization rates with ICSI, was often rationalized as being patient-related; other laboratories considered that it was probably medium-related, but felt that the improvement in embryo development at Day 3 was worth the lower number of embryos obtained. However, since the principles of quality require providing "more," the apparently compromised fertilization rate was seen as a reason for troubleshooting, to determine whether improvements could be made in the number of zygotes obtained from an IVF cycle.

The steps taken in this exercise were the same as those outlined in the troubleshooting flow-chart (Figure 8.1):

There seems to be a problem: An apparently lower-than-expected IVF fertilization rate.

- *Collect data:* Fertilization rates, and the incidence of complete failure of fertilization:
  - For IVF cycles (retrospectively);
  - For contemporaneous IVF and ICSI cycles;
- Embryo quality and cleavage rates (retrospectively).

Analyze data: Review of the fertilization rates and embryo quality

Define the problem(s): (a) The new medium results in better embryo development (not a problem); but
(b) The number of zygotes is reduced for IVF cycles.

Design experiments: (a) *Develop a hypothesis:*

- If the number of zygotes is lower than expected, then is it because gamete function is impaired?:
  - Since the number of zygotes from ICSI is not affected, the oocytes are probably not affected.

- Therefore, maybe sperm function is affected:
  - We know that spermatozoa metabolize glucose (reviewed by Ford and Rees, 1990);
  - We know that glucose is necessary for mouse sperm capacitation and hyperactivation (pre-requisites for zona penetration) (Fraser and Quinn, 1981);
  - But it had been reported that IVF could be achieved successfully in medium without glucose and that the proportion of motile spermatozoa was not affected (Quinn, 1995).
- Therefore – could it be that sperm function is affected, rather than the proportion of motile spermatozoa? In other words, was the *quality*, rather than the *quantity*, of sperm movement being affected?

(b) *Test the hypothesis*: The procedure followed has been presented in detail elsewhere (Mortimer, 2002). However, briefly:

- Semen samples that met the lab's criteria for IVF were used (n = 11).
- The samples were washed as for IVF, using PureSperm gradients.
- The pellets were harvested and re-suspended to 0.5 ml, then divided into two portions.
- 4 ml of medium ± 2.8 mM glucose were added and the sperm suspensions centrifuged.
- Pellets were re-suspended to 0.5 ml in medium ± 2.8 mM glucose (according to treatment group), incubated for 60 minutes in a 6% CO_2 atmosphere.
- Sperm motility was assessed using CASA.

Collect data:

The results showed that while the proportion of motile spermatozoa was unchanged in the incubation period by the presence or absence of glucose, the proportion of hyperactivated spermatozoa *was* significantly reduced in medium that did not contain glucose.

Prioritize problems:

There was only one problem being investigated, that of gamete (sperm) function, so no prioritization was necessary.

Resolve problems:

The problem was with the fertilization rate in low-glucose medium. Since it was apparently solved by the addition of glucose to the same medium, a two-stage medium was created for all clinical IVF cycles. The fertilization medium was the low-glucose medium, supplemented with 2.8 mM glucose, and the cleavage medium was the original low-glucose medium.

Monitor outcome: This had to be done retrospectively:

- The number of IVF cycles with complete failure of fertilization was reduced significantly, and the fertilization rates achieved over all IVF cycles increased significantly.
- The embryo cleavage rate was not affected by the addition of glucose to the fertilization medium.
- But Day 3 embryo morphology was significantly improved.

These outcomes led to the next question: *Could it be that the incubation of gametes in glucose-containing medium confers a developmental advantage?* But since the observation is a positive side-effect of the solution, we're now past troubleshooting and into research...

Troubleshooting an incident

This incident involved the loss of oocytes or embryos belonging to several patients due to a shelf collapsing in an older model incubator. Such a "shelf-collapse" problem is obviously rare, and therefore further explanation for the cause of the problem was sought.

There seems to be a problem: A shelf in an older model incubator collapsed, resulting in the loss of patients' gametes and embryos.

Collect data: Review of the circumstances that led to the shelf collapse.

Analyze data: At inspection, where it was confirmed that the shelf that had collapsed was, indeed, unstable, and that the problem was easily re-created, the following issues were noted:

- In the particular model of incubator involved, the left and right shelf support brackets are fastened to the inside walls of the incubator using knurled nuts at the top and bottom. Two knurled nuts from the top of the left and right shelf support brackets were missing, and another that should have held the bottom of the right-hand bracket was loose. Upon manipulation of the upper shelf the right-hand support bracket came away from the inside of the incubator and both shelves collapsed.
- Inspection of the underside of the upper shelf revealed that the metal runner was to the outside of the shelf support rail, instead of to the inside. As a result the shelf was located several millimeters to the right of its correct location on the support rail, increasing the likelihood that it could fall past the left-hand support rail at the front of the incubator chamber. However, even when the shelf was installed correctly, with both the metal runners located to the inside of the support rails, the shelf could still be coerced to slip past the left-hand support rail at the front of the incubator chamber – whether this was because shelves from another model of incubator had been used, or it was a matter of poor design, remains unknown.

- Large glass desiccators were employed as modular incubators inside the incubator chambers (one on each of the upper and lower shelves) to allow use of a low-oxygen pre-mixed gas. Each desiccator was supplied through a length of highly flexible silicone tubing (which had a "high friction" surface characteristic), passed between the left-hand shelf support brackets and the side of the incubator to prevent them inadvertently knocking against dishes being equilibrated on the shelves outside the desiccators. The presence of these tubes made re-installing the shelves more difficult, since they had to be slid past the tubing; this might have contributed to the risk of their incorrect lateral placement. Also, when attaching and disconnecting the tubing it could easily catch against the left-hand edge of the shelf, and tugging on the tubing could dislodge the shelf to the right, again increasing the risk of the front of the shelf slipping past the support rail.
- During discussions it was discovered that for incubator cleaning hospital policy required that the removable interior components, including the shelves, support brackets, and knurled retaining nuts, be sent to a central washing and sterilization facility. Unfortunately the full complement of nuts was not always returned, and the lab "made do" with what they had.

Clearly the shelf-collapse incident was due, in large part, to the incorrect re-installation of the shelf support brackets (the two missing and one loose knurled nuts) and incorrect replacement of the shelf with regard to the location of its right-hand runner and the shelf support rail. The concomitant use of modular incubators obviously increased the opportunity for the incident to occur because of their weight and the presence of the gassing tubing.

Define the problem(s):	Unfortunately, this already unlikely incident was actually compounded to become more of a disaster because the incubator in question – one of three culture incubators in the laboratory – actually contained all the current patients' oocytes and embryos.
Design experiments:	Review the circumstances that led to all of the patients' oocytes and embryos being cultured in only one of the incubators.
Collect data:	The shelf collapse incident occurred on a Friday. According to the lab's regular schedule one incubator was cleaned, and its CO_2 control system reset, each week on the Thursday. Unfortunately, due to a shortage of embryologists in comparison to the caseload on the day before the incident occurred, it was decided to delay the incubator cleaning until the following day. On the Friday, the incubator was taken out of service (so only two incubators were available for culture) and cleaned, but then, working in haste, the wrong incubator's

CO_2 re-calibration button was pressed. Fortunately this mistake was recognized immediately, but, nevertheless, all cases had to be moved into a single working culture incubator – and that was when the shelf collapsed.

Prioritize problems: Obviously the incident, and especially its ultimate magnitude, must be considered to have occurred as a result of an exceptional set of circumstances! Underlying the more technical issues, both the established under-staffing of the IVF laboratory and the concomitants of the policy for central sterilization of incubator shelving systems were also root causes in the genesis of this incident – but these more general issues cannot excuse not having spare retaining nuts, and incorrect re-assembly of the incubator shelves.

Resolve problems: Changes in policy:

- Reduce the incidence of understaffing;
- Ensure availability of necessary spare parts;

Staff education:

- Incubator cleaning procedure;
- Recommissioning of incubator after cleaning process.

Monitor outcome: The problem did not recur.

Troubleshooting a maintenance process

In the previous examples, following the troubleshooting process as presented in Figure 8.1 was key to identifying and understanding the problem. However, in a situation where the issue is primarily organizational or administrative in nature, it is not always necessary – or perhaps practical – to include every step in sequence. In the following example, the "error" was simply one of timing, rather than something that required data to establish its basis.

A well-managed, accredited IVF lab sent one of its two Cook MINC incubators to the regular third-party service agent for its annual preventative maintenance. The incubator was duly returned and, as per the lab's standard maintenance schedule, the lab then shipped the second incubator off for servicing. Unfortunately, in the rush to get the second incubator off, perhaps due to impending severe winter weather or simple forgetfulness, the lab had omitted to verify the proper operation of the first incubator on-site before sending away the second – even though this was current policy.

Fortunately, before re-introducing the MINC back into clinical use the incubator's temperature was checked using a dummy culture dish and thermocouple (which had been previously calibrated in-house against a certified reference thermometer), and it was discovered that the temperature of the incubation chambers was only 35.5–35.8°C. Unfortunately, the service report did not include a copy of the certificate of calibration for the device(s) used by the service engineer to perform the re-calibration post-servicing (as expected under ISO 15189:2012 ¶4.13(I)), and direct communication with the engineer was initiated.

Discussions with the service company identified that the particular temperature measuring devices used when checking temperatures during servicing were not adjustable, and therefore corrections had to be applied to each measurement, based on in-house calibrations performed using a Hart Temperature Calibrator. The conclusion was that the service probes appeared to have varied since their previous calibration, and hence the offsets applied were no longer correct.

In response to this issue:

- The service company has since implemented a procedural change to verify the calibration of their service probes at the time of each job; and
- The lab has added formal documentation of incubator performance verification after servicing, and requires that this must be completed before another incubator can be taken out of routine operation.

Basically, all that is required for effective troubleshooting is the ability to go through all the aspects of the perceived problem in an organized way. However, there is an inescapable need for a thorough knowledge of the basic science that underlies the field, as well as a moderate understanding of practical considerations that affect how we do things in the IVF lab. This latter need encompasses a broad range of areas of practical knowledge, including, for example, various aspects of engineering as they relate to equipment design and operation. Clearly being a good IVF scientist, and especially an IVF lab director, requires a great deal more of one than just being a skilled embryologist – and this is the basis of the standard accreditation requirement for being a "learning organization." Education is a lifelong process and as you become more senior there is a concomitant need for broader knowledge that includes many areas that might previously have seemed extraneous or superfluous to being a good embryologist.

Risk management: being proactive

Risk management is all about being proactive. Risk analysis is undertaken to identify where things might go wrong. This does require some experience and, indeed, the wider your experience the more likely you are to be able to recognize issues as problems or to identify potential problems. The general principles of risk management are described in *ISO 31000:2009 Risk Management – Principles and guidelines*, and will be discussed later in this chapter. A simple overview can also be found in Hobbs (2009).

"Why bother with that? It's never happened here!"

How often have you identified a potential problem, only to be told "Oh that's never been a problem here" or "We've never had a problem with that," or "Why waste our time, that's just so unlikely." Of course, the truth is that this head-in-the-sand mentality is exactly why some of the worst problems in IVF labs have arisen. We have personally experienced situations where an identified risk was pooh-poohed by the medical director, general manager or equivalent, only to have just that problem occur a few weeks later – although professional confidentiality clearly precludes quoting specific examples! The dreaded "It's never happened here ..." should probably be considered a warning bell that a proper risk assessment should be undertaken forthwith. After all, Captain Edward John Smith hadn't hit any icebergs before the maiden voyage of the Titanic, either!

Can we eliminate risk?

Of course, everyone would like to believe that we can eliminate all risk from our laboratories, but in reality we must consider things in practical terms and recognize that different risks are amenable to different levels of resolution.

Risk elimination

There are a few risks that we can eliminate from our IVF labs, e.g. banning the wearing of perfume and aftershave to reduce the level of VOCs.

Risk avoidance

In risk management terms, risk avoidance is used to describe an informed decision not to become involved in activities that lead to the possibility of the risk being realized. Prohibiting smoking in an area where there are flammable, volatile solvents is a good example of risk avoidance. An extreme example of risk avoidance in the "real world" is shown in Figure 9.1.

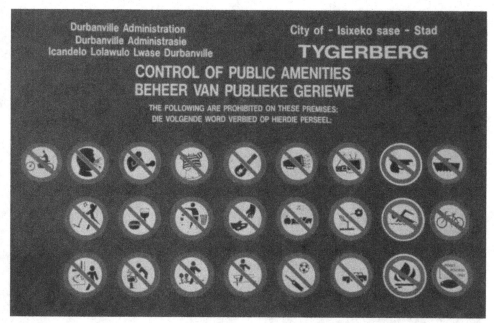

Figure 9.1 A rather extreme example of risk avoidance. The sign was photographed by DM in a suburban park in Cape Town, South Africa.

Risk reduction or risk minimization

These terms are essentially synonymous and are used in risk management to describe the application of appropriate techniques to reduce the likelihood of an adverse event, its consequences, or both. A real-world example of this type of action is shown in Figure 9.2. In the IVF lab, the management of the cryobank is a good area to see risk minimization strategies: not only should the cryotanks' usage of liquid nitrogen be monitored on a regular basis (e.g. their level at weekly top-up for tanks not fitted with an autofill system) but they must also be connected to low-level alarms in case of tank failure, especially outside normal working hours. Further dimensions of risk minimization in this example are the maintenance of a spare cryotank, partially filled with liquid nitrogen, ready to receive specimens from a suspect cryotank, or the "split storage" of each patient's specimens between two separate cryotanks. Risk reduction/minimization is discussed in some detail later in this chapter.

Risk transfer

This is a risk management concept that describes the shifting of the burden of the risk to another party. Probably (hopefully!) the most common example of risk transfer in an IVF lab is insurance.

Risk acceptance or risk retention

This risk management term is used to describe an informed decision to accept the consequences and likelihood of a particular risk (e.g. the possibility of a meteor strike, discussed in Chapter 4).

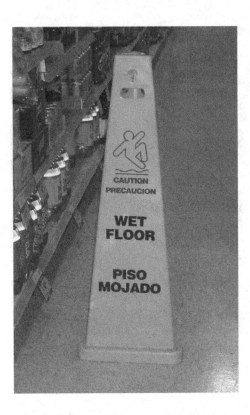

Figure 9.2 A common example of risk minimization.

How do we manage risk?

An interesting illustration of how risk management typically uses several strategies to achieve a comprehensive solution is that of fire (Figure 9.3).

We have fire insurance so that if our premises are damaged or lost due to fire we will be recompensed and be able to repair or rebuild. But while such an event would be disastrous for us professionally, as well as personally, it could be even worse for the patients. That is why we also have fire drills to evacuate the premises in case of a serious fire, fire extinguishers to put out any fires that might occur before they can do much damage, and fire alarms to alert us that a fire has started. Even so, we could suffer appreciable financial loss during repairs, or loss of professional confidence that leads to a drop-off in referrals, a fall in workload, and hence a down-sizing of the program with all that this entails. Therefore, it is wise that we also have fire prevention to try and avoid a fire occurring in the first place.

This overall scheme might seem somewhat redundant, but it is really an example of strategic planning – we should look at its components in reverse order:

- Fire prevention as an expression of risk avoidance: we avoid doing things or creating situations that increase the risk of fire, e.g. by refraining from smoking in areas where there are solvents, storing solvents in proper flammables cabinets, and ensuring that electrical equipment is properly wired.
- Fire extinguishers to reduce the amount of damage that a fire can do.
- Fire alarms, to make sure that we get as much warning as possible of a fire, so as to use a fire extinguisher sooner, or have more time to evacuate staff, patients, and data backups.

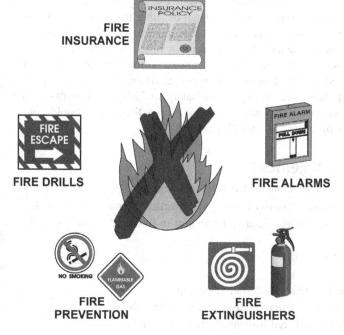

Figure 9.3 An illustration of the multifaceted approach usually taken towards fire; embracing various risk avoidance, risk prevention, risk minimization, and risk transfer features.

- Fire drills to make evacuations more efficient.
- Fire insurance as the last resort to allow us to rebuild and/or recompense as effectively as possible.

This sort of multilayered strategy should be applied throughout the IVF center, including the laboratory, or, indeed, any workplace.

Risk reduction

Rather like the quality cycle (see Chapter 3), risk reduction is an iterative process that never reaches perfection. While we can reach an asymptotic state where all controllable risks have been avoided, eliminated, or controlled to the best of our abilities, the exclusion of all risk – "perfection" in this sense – is not a realistic goal. In the real world, constraints will be applied to this process, for example:

- Cost–benefit scenarios, usually determined at the corporate level;
- Physical limitations, e.g. available space for back-up facilities, such as spare incubators or cryogenic storage tanks; and
- Shortage of trained staff to ensure necessary "slack" in the system (see Chapter 4).

Taking responsibility

As professionals, we all must accept responsibility for our actions. This subject was considered in the discussion on identifying "high risk" IVF laboratories in Chapter 4, but it is such an important aspect that it will be re-iterated here.

When a team member does not take enough care to ensure that they have performed – and completed – all the tasks that were assigned to them it can be either intentional or unintentional. In either case it is unprofessional behavior, but at least if it is unintentional it is only an expression of inadequate or incomplete training, a problem for which there should be an easy remedy. The intentional omission of parts of one's job can only continue without jeopardizing outcomes if there are others who take the time (and/or are prepared to make the time) to ensure that the whole process is completed: in effect they are the "safety net." All professionals must be prepared to work without a safety net; if someone cannot do this then (s)he should not be working in an IVF laboratory or, indeed, in an IVF center.

The benefits of risk management

The following benefits will ensue from an effective risk management program:

- Better knowledge of the process, thereby helping to eliminate the need for re-work;
- More efficient processes and systems, leading to savings in time and resources, and hence money;
- Reduced stress levels for the staff;
- Reduced risk of error;
- Higher quality of service and hence customer satisfaction;
- Reduced legal implications, and hence reduced potential for liability;
- Lower risk rating can lead to reduced insurance premiums; and
- Documented organizational history.

Basically, poorly designed processes or ones vulnerable to failure are targeted for replacement by better-designed processes; existing processes also benefit by virtue of introducing improvements before adverse events occur. Properly conducted and documented FMEAs record the evolution of the laboratory's processes. This should prevent past mistakes from being repeated, e.g. by well-intentioned but inexperienced staff, and will enable new employees to learn the laboratory's systems and their operational characteristics more rapidly.

Developing a risk management program

Like an effective quality management system, a successful risk management program must be integrated into all levels of the organization. Clearly, therefore, a risk management program must include the whole IVF center – restricting it just to the laboratory is short-sighted and will severely limit its total benefits to the center. After establishing the extent (scope) and purpose (goals) of the risk management program, an individual or team should be designated and assigned responsibility for its development and implementation.

Seven general principles create a framework within which effective risk management can be accomplished.

1. *Global perspective:* Consider the IVF center's development within the context of the "industry" – competing centers (getting results, referrals, etc.), government regulations, licensing, accreditation, etc. Recognize the potential value of opportunity, but also the potential impact of adverse effects.
2. *Forward-looking view:* Always look to the future. Identify uncertainties and anticipate potential adverse outcomes.

3. *Open communication:* Encourage and facilitate formal, informal, and impromptu communication and the free flow of information at and between all areas and levels of the center. Always value the individual voice: anyone can contribute unique knowledge and insight that can help identify or manage risk.

4. *Integrated management:* Make risk management an integral part of the center's activities.

5. *Continuous process:* Like the quality cycle, risk management is a never-ending process.

6. *Shared vision:* Build a vision of quality of service and care throughout the center based on common purpose and shared ownership; focus on results.

7. *Teamwork:* Everyone in the center must work cooperatively towards common goals. No-one knows everything, so knowledge, skills and talents should be shared among all members of staff.

Anyone who has experience of a formal laboratory accreditation will recognize these seven principles as core elements of the process. For an IVF center the ultimate goal of risk management is to reduce the likelihood of having to expend resources on dealing with catastrophic incidents – resources that will probably not be readily available when needed. This is why proactive risk management is so important, and why familiarity with the fundamental concepts and tools used in risk management should be an essential part of the training for all scientists working in IVF labs.

Although the widely accepted joint Australia/New Zealand standard for developing a risk management program AS/NZS 4360:1999 has been replaced by ISO 31000:2009 *Risk Management – Principles and Guidelines,* the outline of the steps involved in the overall process of developing a risk management program that it contained was particularly clear, and was the basis for Table 9.1 and illustrated in Figure 9.4.

The *risk register* is the centralized archive of all documentation pertaining to an organization's management of its identified risks.

Illustrative examples of risk management in the IVF lab

The following examples have not been presented in the strict format of formal risk analyses, but rather as explanations of the issues and how each IVF center should go about evaluating and managing the risks for themselves.

Off-site collection of sperm samples

Even though it is better for any number of reasons that the semen sample to be washed for use in IVF or IUI is produced on-site at the clinic, it often happens that the man produces it elsewhere and it is brought to the clinic by the woman. While in virtually all cases it could be correctly assumed by the clinic staff that the semen is from the woman's partner, this is not always so. There have been incidents in which a woman has brought someone else's semen to the clinic, without her partner's knowledge. To avoid the litigation and adverse publicity that might eventuate from such cases, the IVF lab needs to have a procedure in place in which the woman warrants that the semen is that of her partner. Similarly, if the man brings the sample to the lab, he should attest formally that it is his. An example of the type of form one could use for this purpose is given in Figure 9.5.

Table 9.1 Major elements of a risk management plan based on the provisions of the now superseded AS/NZS 4360.

Plan element	Explanation
General	Establish the purpose of the plan and embed the risk management process into all the organization's processes (this should be the primary objective of the plan).
Ensure support of senior management	Without this any risk management is foredoomed.
Develop the risk management policy	Defining and documenting the organization's policy, including management's commitment to it, is essential.
Communicate the policy	Create an infrastructure to ensure that managing risk becomes embedded throughout the organization's processes and into its culture.
Establish accountability and authority	Create the framework for delegated personnel to build and implement the plan under the aegis of senior management.
Customize the risk management process	Interpret and apply the standard to create the organization's risk management processes, including specifying measures of its performance and criteria for judging its success.
Resourcing	Identifying and allocating adequate resources is vital for the success of the plan.
Organizational level risk management plan	An integrated plan for managing risk at all levels of the organization must be developed and implemented, including its incorporation into all the organization's processes and systems.
Manage risks at the area, project, and team levels	Plans for each subordinate area within the organization must be developed and implemented; these plans must be consistent with, and integrated into, the organizational level plan.
Monitor and review	Risks are not static so risk management must be a dynamic process.

Disposal of frozen embryos

Frozen embryos are held for a couple's possible future attempts at pregnancy. It is standard that the embryos are considered to belong to the couple, and that any decision as to their disposition must be agreed to by both people. However, how the couple notifies the IVF center of their wishes, particularly when it is to donate the embryos, or to discard them, can have important ramifications. For example, one center might consider that if one partner calls the clinic and says that the couple wishes to have their embryos discarded, this is good enough to order the lab to dispose of the frozen embryos – not considering that this might not be the wish of both partners and thereby exposing itself to the risk of litigation, as well as causing significant distress to the unwilling partner. Another center might follow the protocol that following the phone call, information regarding the options for disposal of the embryos (for informed consent) is sent to the couple's last known address, along with a "request to dispose of frozen embryos" form that requires the couple's wishes to be expressed explicitly, and that has to be signed by both partners with each signature witnessed by a third party. Alternatively, it might require that both partners attend a counselling session at the center

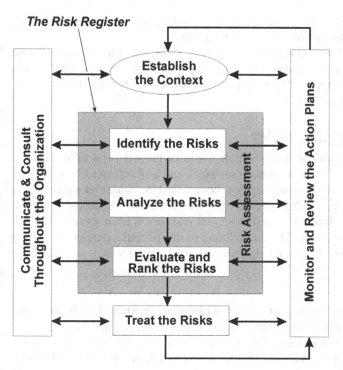

The Risk Register

Figure 9.4 A diagrammatic representation of the risk management process, based on the provisions of the now superseded AS/NSZ 4360 (see also ISO 31000:2009).

THE XYZ FERTILITY CENTRE

RELEASE FOR SEMEN SAMPLES PRODUCED OFF–SITE

If sample delivered to the Lab by self:

I,_____confirm that
(Name: LAST, First)
the semen sample that I have delivered to The XYZ

Fertility Centre today_____ is my own
(Date)
semen, produced off-site.

LABORATORY USE ONLY

Lab Accession No.   **A0**___ –_____
Date of sample: ___ / _____ / 200__
Time received by Lab: ___ : ____hrs
XFC Chart No.   _____

Signed : _____

If sample delivered to the Lab by partner or family member:

I,_____ confirm that the semen sample that I have delivered to The XYZ Fertility
(Name: LAST, First)

Centre today_____ is the semen of my husband / partner,_____,
(Date)   *(Name: LAST, First)*

which was produced off-site.   Signed :_____

FRM-XFCLab012-20040324 Off-site release

Figure 9.5 An example of an off-site sperm sample form that can be used to manage risk in the IVF lab.

before signing the form. This center might also allow a "cooling off" period after the receipt of the completed form, in case the couple change their mind.

By considering the risks involved in handling a request to dispose of frozen embryos, the second IVF center has done all it can to ensure that both partners' opinions are heard. Apart from reducing the exposure of the center to litigation, it is also a more respectful approach that adheres to the principles of quality.

Parallel processing of sperm samples

Often in a busy lab, more than one sperm sample has to be prepared at a time. This has enormous potential for disaster (i.e. mixing up samples), and a system must be developed that addresses this. Apart from the witnessing that should take place whenever a specimen is moved from one container to another (see "Tools versus solutions" in Chapter 5), there should be policies and procedures in place that prevent one person from actually manipulating more than one sample at once. A good solution to this potential problem is to have separate test tube racks to isolate the materials for each case (Figure 9.6).

Labelling OPU tubes

It is a standard accreditation requirement, and good laboratory practice, that all containers holding a patient's tissues and fluids be labelled (ideally with two unique identifiers; see Figure 5.11). An example of where this may not be followed in some IVF labs is in the labelling of the OPU tubes. If the IVF center is one in which there is always a 30–60 minute gap between oocyte retrievals, then the management might not consider this risk to be very

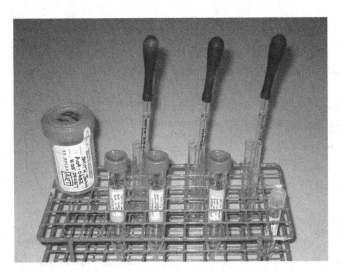

Figure 9.6 A system to minimize the risk of cross-contamination between sperm specimens being processed in parallel. All the tubes, etc., for a given specimen are placed in a single rack so that even if two specimens are being centrifuged together, they are each harvested and re-suspended separately. Note that the semen collection jar is labelled with the man's name and the andrology lab reference number (A04–0682) as well as the date and time of collection. Each tube and pipette are labelled with the name plus both the andrology lab number and the oocyte retrieval case number (R04–0179) as identifiers, along with the date and the purpose of each item. There is no label on the rack because it is the identity of each of the individual items that must be verified at each stage of the process; if there was a large label on the rack there might be a tendency to read only that when going to work on a sample.

great. However, if the center is a very busy one, with many oocyte retrievals in a day, and very short lag times between cases, then the management might see the risk of mis-identification of oocytes as significant, and insist upon a labelling procedure.

Therefore, the decision as to whether non-labelling of OPU tubes constitutes a risk (i.e. mixing tubes between patients) is one that must be addressed by each IVF center individually. However, labelling each container would seem to be a prudent risk minimization strategy.

Temperature control during oocyte retrieval

Because of the meiotic spindle the oocyte is exquisitely temperature-sensitive. Cooling causes de-polymerization of the spindle (Pickering et al., 1990; Almeida and Bolton, 1995; Wang et al., 2001), releasing the chromosomes into the ooplasm. Although the spindle re-polymerizes upon warming, there is considered to be a significant risk that one or more chromosomes might not become re-attached to the spindle and hence a state of aneuploidy would be created at the second meiotic division, which occurs in response to the spermatozoon activating the oocyte at fertilization. It has been hypothesized that repeated cycles of warming and cooling during oocyte retrieval might increase the risk of aneuploidy in human embryos, and hence the degree to which an IVF lab's systems protect the oocyte from such stresses might be at least a partial explanation of the differences in embryo aneuploidy rates reported by various centers. Anecdotally, in the multicenter study of treatment-related chromosome abnormalities in human embryos published by Munné et al. (1997), the center with the lowest observed rate of aneuploidy was the only one using an IVF chamber workstation (see Chapter 11).

The following list enumerates the factors that can contribute to the cooling of oocytes during the OPU procedure ("warm" means at or as close as possible to, 37 °C, and "cold" refers to <35 °C):

- Empty OPU tubes are not kept warm;
- Flush buffer is not pre-warmed prior to use;
- Pre-warmed flush buffer is allowed to cool during use;
- Follicular fluid is not kept warm during aspiration into the collection tubes;
- Workstation heated surface not properly calibrated to maintain the "egg search" dish contents at 37 °C;
- Cooling effect of the air flow during egg search (a major problem in laminar air flow cabinets where it is ambient temperature air), which is exacerbated by using larger diameter dishes and taking longer to search for COCs;
- Holding COCs in a glass pipette for longer than absolutely necessary during their handling and washing (exacerbated by ambient temperature air flow);
- Washing or holding medium not kept warm during the egg search procedure; and
- Bicarbonate-buffered washing or holding medium not kept under an appropriate CO_2-enriched atmosphere during the egg search procedure (therefore should use an appropriate HEPES- or MOPS-buffered medium).

The problem of maintaining temperature throughout the OPU and egg search procedure is an excellent illustration that not only do perceived problems represent opportunities for improvement, but that if a known negative factor is recognized in a system then one's effort is far better spent on minimizing it (ideally, eliminating it) than trying to prove whether or not it's actually a significant factor in your particular circumstance. The latter principle can be considered as the tempering of scientific method with common sense – there is no point

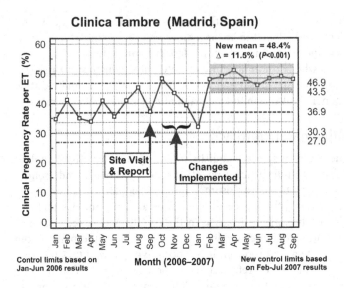

Figure 9.7 Illustration of the beneficial effects of improving temperature control during the OPU procedure and the handling of oocytes.

proving that a known deleterious factor (in this case cooling oocytes, risking spindle depolymerization) is actually affecting your results, just eliminate it and thereby exclude it from both current and future concerns!

Having said this, it should be noted that this is one of the most insidious problems we see in labs that we visit. We are indebted to Dr Rocío Nuñez Calonge, lab director and quality manager at the Clínica Tambre in Madrid for allowing us to show the data contained in Figure 9.7. After visiting the Tambre lab in September 2006, a series of recommendations were made to make changes that would reduce the opportunity for cooling of COCs during the OPU and egg search procedure, and during handling of oocytes and embryos in general. After implementing these changes the clinical pregnancy rate per ET (across all patients) increased significantly from 36.9% (with month-to-month control limits of 27.0 to 46.9%, i.e. ±10%) to 48.4% with control limits of around ±5%. This pattern of improvement is typical of an improved process: an increase in the overall level of success combined with a decrease in its variability.

Packaging systems for cryobanking gametes and embryos

Of great current concern to those working in human gamete and embryo cryobanking are issues arising from concerns over the risk of contamination either by other specimens in the same cryotank or by contaminated liquid nitrogen. Even though such an occurrence has never been reported for sperm or embryos, and the risk is generally accepted to be vanishingly small, it does represent a finite risk and all reasonable measures should be taken to reduce the chance of its occurring (see the discussion concerning this issue in Chapter 4).

A further dimension to resolving this issue is the ability to achieve the "correct" cooling and warming curves during freezing and thawing within the physical constraints of the various packaging devices, especially the vexed and persistent argument of straws versus cryovials.

Both these matters were considered some years ago within a general framework of risk analysis and management, utilizing the available evidence and perceptions of "best practice" from both the medical and legal perspectives (Mortimer, 2004b; using technical and biological information reviewed in Mortimer, 2004a). Table 9.2 illustrates a formal risk

Table 9.2 An example of using FMEA to evaluate the safety of cryostorage packaging devices for gametes and embryos. "R" = the risk rating or consequence of the risk happening, "L" = the likelihood of the risk occurring and "C" = the calculated "criticality" of the risk (C= RxL). *Denotes conditions assuming a device is used correctly according to the manufacturer's instructions, and †identifies situations where it is assumed that best practice laboratory procedure has been followed. For numeric superscripts see Notes, below. Reproduced from Mortimer (2004b) with permission.

Risk	Consequence				IMV 0.25-ml straw		IMV 0.50-ml straw		CBS High Security Straw	
			Cryovial							
	Description of failure	R	L	C	L	C	L	C	L	C
Contamination of the outside of the device during filling	Will carry contamination into the cryogenic storage vessel	4	7	**28**	8†	**32**	8†	**32**	0*	**0**
Microbial transmission through the device wall	Risk of outward contamination of cryogenic storage vessel or inward contamination of specimen	4	1	**4**	1	**4**	1	**4**	0*	**0**
Fragility of the device at −196°C	Risk of breakage during handling while in storage (e.g. audits)	7	0	**0**	3†1	**21**	2†1	**14**	0*	**0**
2° containment needed for safe use of device under "extreme" storage conditions (i.e. −196°C)	Ability to provide reasonable expectation of hermetic integrity of the specimen	6	9*	**54**	4†	**24**	4†	**24**	0*	**0**
Adverse practical sequelae of the 2° containment system	Handling difficulties in attaching devices to canes	5	5*	**25**	0	**0**	0	**0**	0*	**0**
Cooling curve of the specimen does not follow the programmed rate closely	Proper cooling rate is not experienced by the specimen, or rate is variable throughout the specimen	7	8	**56**	1	**7**	2	**14**	2	**14**
Warming rate of specimen does not follow ambient temperature closely during thawing	Proper (rapid) warming rate cannot be achieved during thawing	6	6†	**36**	1†	**6**	2†	**12**	2†	**12**

Table 9.2 (cont.)

Risk	Consequence	Cryovial			IMV 0.25-ml straw		IMV 0.50-ml straw		CBS High Security Straw	
	Description of failure	R	L	C	L	C	L	C	L	C
Risk of inadvertent warming during handling of cryobanked device	Risk of ice re-crystallization due to specimen warming above the glass transition temperature of water (ca. −132°C)	7	2	**14**	$6^{†2}$	**42**	$4^{†2}$	**28**	$4^{†2}$	**28**
Explosion hazard when thawing specimen	Explosive over-pressure due to evaporation of liquid nitrogen trapped inside the device	5	$4^†$	**20**	$2^†$	**10**	$2^†$	**10**	0*	**0**
ID information can be lost or smudged during cryostorage	Integrity of identifying information of each unit stored	8	1	**8**	$2^†$	**16**	$1^†$	**8**	$0^{*†}$	**0**
Total criticality scores				**245**		**162³**		**146³**		**54³**

Notes:
[1] These risk likelihood ratings reflect the typical practice in many human IVF cryobanks of storing straws in narrow visotubes attached to canes, rather than according to the manufacturer's instructions to store straws in visotubes that are kept inside goblets in canisters (which would merit reducing these ratings by 1 rank). When attached to canes there is the possibility of (inadvertent) attempted flexion of the straws during their removal from the visotubes.
[2] These risk likelihood ratings reflect the typical practice in many human IVF cryobanks of handling straws in isolation, rather than inside visotubes where the surrounding LN₂ would guarantee their remaining at −196°C. If, as per the manufacturer's recommendations, straws were only handled in visotubes (except when removing for thawing) these risk likelihood ratings could be reduced to values of 1.
[3] If the correct practices described in Notes 1 and 2 were followed, these total criticality scores would be reduced to 113, 118, and 33 respectively.

analysis, in the format of an FMEA, performed on the four most common packaging devices used for cryopreserving human gametes and embryos, and leads to the clear conclusion that the High Security Straws from CryoBio System (Paris, France) represent the current best practice from the perspectives of not only the technical achievement of cryopreservation but also biocontainment.

With the widespread conversion to vitrification for oocytes and embryos, the issue of possible cross-contamination during cryostorage has re-surfaced. Although some experts simply declare that it is of no concern, the simple fact that some regulatory agencies are concerned about such a possibility means it cannot be ignored. This means that open packaging devices for vitrification, which have generally been accepted due to the high success rates that can be achieved using them, will come under increasing threat from closed devices, and even more so from sealed devices – especially those that have established biocontainment – as their equivalent efficacy is established (e.g. Van Landuyt et al., 2011; Stoop et al., 2012).

The rapid adoption of vitrification has also generated more general recognition of the risk of inadvertent specimen warming during cryostorage, since devices that hold ultra-micro volume specimens have minute thermal mass, making them highly temperature labile. This means that the inadvertent exposure of such a specimen to temperatures above the ice transition point of water (i.e. above −132°C) for even a very few seconds can lead to ice re-crystallization and hence cellular damage.

Monitoring storage cryotanks

Everyone knows that storage cryotanks need to be topped-up regularly, but the degree of care paid to these critical pieces of equipment is often rather lackadaisical heading towards totally unconcerned – after all, how often have you had a problem with one? We have experienced three tanks that have shown signs of failure, and fortunately none that have actually failed with specimens inside them. The first was back in the 1980s when an andrology lab technician commented that he was sure that a particular tank seemed to need more LN_2 to fill it up each week (tanks were filled religiously every Friday afternoon) than the others. The response was to have him measure the levels before re-filling the tanks, and compare them over a few weeks. Sure enough the suspect tank was requiring more LN_2 to top it up – and the amount was slowly increasing week by week. So the tank was replaced with a new one and the specimens transferred across without any loss or damage. Measuring the level of the remaining LN_2 in each tank before it was filled each week then became standard practice – and since it was hard to see a pattern in a series of numbers we thought to plot them on graph paper to see any trends (remember graph paper? – this was before Excel...!).

This practice was maintained in other labs and, over the years, we identified two other tanks that showed similar patterns of behavior – and replaced each of them as quickly as possible and avoided any adverse outcomes. Overall, the procedure that we adopted from these experiences can be summarized quite simply:

- Fill tanks at a specific regular interval, one which will allow for sufficient evaporative loss of LN_2, but not enough to be any concern for the specimens stored in the tank. Some labs insist that they must fill tanks two or even three times per week, but with static holding times running at several to many weeks this is clearly unnecessary. For example, a Taylor Wharton HC35 dewar has a static holding time of 130 days, based on an evaporative loss rate of 0.27 liters of LN_2 per day, and a rated "working time" of 81 days – i.e. 11.5 weeks at typical access rates.
- Measure and log the level of the remaining LN_2 before topping up the tank.
- Fill the tank to a standard level each time – but this does not mean over-fill it and spray out excess LN_2 when replacing the insulated plug. In fact this is not only dangerous to yourself and others, it's also bad for the tank (see "Cryotank abuse", below).
- Finally, in order to identify when a trend in the data plot becomes a cause for concern, we now use control chart principles to create warning and control limits for the pre-topping-up LN_2 level. Simply calculate the mean and standard deviation of a series of measurements, e.g. over a six-month period, and use the mean −2SD value as a warning that the tank is behaving abnormally, and the mean −3SD level as evidence that the tank is now behaving abnormally (see Figure 9.8). Of course incidents like having to search for a lost straw, an unusually high number of tank accesses over the preceding

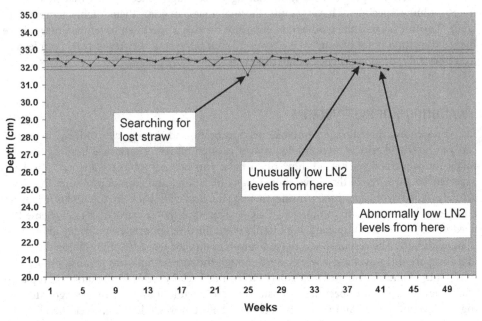

Figure 9.8 Illustration of how process control charts can be used for the effective monitoring of liquid nitrogen (LN₂) usage by storage cryotanks. In this imaginary example, control mean and warning/control limits were based on historical data collected during 2008 (measurements of the LN₂ level before each weekly re-fill of the tank). While the transitory dip in week 28 was explained by having to search for a lost straw, by week 39 the gradual decline in remaining LN₂ level has crossed the warning limit, establishing real cause for concern that the tank was performing abnormally, and by week 41 it had crossed the control limit – at which point the tank was deemed unusable.

week (e.g. due to transferring a large number of straws from the tank), or a tank audit, will lead to unusually low LN₂ levels and must be flagged as abnormal events.

Maintaining a spare cryotank is an important element of any IVF lab's risk management system. This tank should be maintained cold, but obviously not full of LN₂ – otherwise when you need it there's no room to put any specimens into it, and the first thing you have to do is dump much of the LN₂! Ideally you should always use the same configuration of tanks so that the canisters can be simply, and directly, moved to another tank. If a tank is in danger of failing, the last thing you want to have to do is start moving all the specimens individually into canisters of a different size. So good cryobank management practice is to have all the tanks of the same model and configuration (at least in terms of canisters), and keep a spare tank ⅓–½ full of LN₂ without its canisters. Many accreditation schemes include this aspect in their surveys, and the UK's HFEA requires maintaining a spare tank as a licensing condition.

Cryotank alarms: What happens if a tank fails outside normal working hours? Fitting a low level and/or high temperature alarm to each storage cryotank is another key element to any risk management system, and these alarms must be connected to a dial-out system so that laboratory staff members are notified of a problem. After all, there's no point in having an alarm going off all night with no-one around to hear it. At the most basic level we have used the Gordinier model 661 combined low level/high temperature sensor/alarm units,

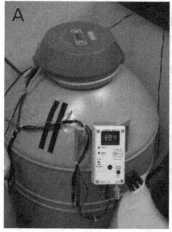
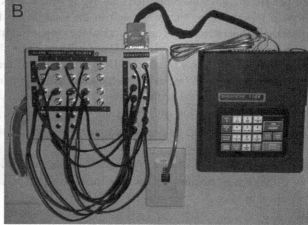

Figure 9.9 Illustrations of equipment for monitoring cryotanks on a real-time basis. In **A** the tank is fitted with a Gordinier model 661 combined liquid nitrogen and temperature sensor that is connected to a Sensaphone dial-out alarm system which is shown in **B**.

connected to a Sensaphone autodialler (see Figure 9.9) for many years. More recently we have used temperature sensors connected to Planer's *ReAssure* system to provide 24/7 monitoring of cryostorage tanks.

Cryotank Failure: What causes a dewar vessel to fail? Obviously the loss of vacuum between the outer and inner vessels reduces the insulation capacity, leading to increased evaporative loss of LN_2 per unit time. But how does loss of vacuum occur?

Catastrophic failure is when the vacuum is lost suddenly, e.g. due to the outer vessel being punctured, or the neck weld failing completely. Fortunately, neither of us has ever seen this as it would, indeed, be a catastrophic event. Imagine a tank holding, say, 35 liters of LN_2 that suddenly boils from liquid to gas – with the accompanied almost 700-fold increase in volume... One would most definitely not want to be a witness to that!

Slow failure is the more typical problem seen with storage dewars, as noted above.

Cryotank Abuse: So how do cryotanks, typically aluminum-walled dewar vessels, lose their vacuum?

Punctures of the outer vessel are extremely rare, but all tanks have a location where there is a protruding metal nipple or other fitting from where the air was evacuated after welding the outer and inner tanks together. These protuberances are protected from mechanical insult by a welded-on cover, but a significant mechanical insult can knock this cover off, and subsequent physical damage could break the seal.

Over-filling a cryotank with LN_2 and then causing the excess LN_2 to overflow the neck when replacing the insulated plug is not only dangerous to yourself and others, it's also bad for the tank. Running LN_2 over the weld between the inner and outer vessels, which is at the rim of the neck, exposes it to repeated cycles of severe cooling and re-warming back to ambient temperature. This stresses the weld (metal fatigue), and even a microscopic crack can lead to a slow loss of vacuum.

Inertial stress is caused by sudden movement, or a sudden stopping of movement, of a cryotank. Consider the construction of a dewar vessel. The inner vessel is full of specimens and LN_2, so in a HC35 tank it will weigh around 35 kg. This inner vessel is, in effect, suspended in a vacuum supported only by the weld at the top of its neck. So the inertia of a sudden movement or stop will result in the inner vessel trying to swing inside the outer vessel, exerting lateral force on the neck of the vessel. Picking up a dewar and then putting it back on the floor in a non-gentle manner will also cause similar stress in a (latero-)vertical direction. While a large insult could cause cracking of the weld, repeated smaller stresses will weaken the metal (metal fatigue), eventually leading to cracking.

Moving Cryotanks: For the reasons discussed above the following principles must be employed when working with cryogenic storage dewars:

- Ideally keep storage tanks in a permanent location, to minimize the need to move them at all.
- When topping-up storage cryotanks, take the supply dewar to the storage dewar.
- If tanks must be moved then have them on roller bases and move them slowly and carefully.

Verification of specimen identity

It is obvious good practice that every time a specimen is labelled, or moved from one container to another, identity checks must be followed strictly, and verified either by a competent human witness, or some validated process or technological solution. Indeed, such practice is mandatory in the UK for a clinic to be licensed by the HFEA. However, verbal double-checking – often referred to as "double witnessing," although there is actually only one person acting as witness, and so the term "witnessing" is correct – might not always produce the benefit expected (see discussion in Brison *et al.*, 2004). Of particular concern is the problem of "involuntary automaticity" (Toft and Mascie-Taylor, 2005), whereby a process that is repetitive becomes automatic and is not carried out properly. In addition, when another member of lab staff has to act as a human witness either (s)he will have to break off what (s)he is doing to go over and perform the specimen verification check, or else the other person will need to wait until (s)he is ready. In either situation there is clearly not only the risk of potential compromise to the gametes or embryos that are either waiting to be verified, or that are left while verifying others elsewhere in the lab, but also possible risks due to loss of focus, forgetfulness, and perhaps even physical loss as a result of careless movement.

Obviously it is the responsibility of the medical director overall, and the lab director in particular for IVF lab processes, to eliminate or at least minimize any opportunity for risk. Consequently, a formal risk assessment of specimen provenance and identification processes should be undertaken to ensure that the risk of specimen mis-identification or confusion ("mix-up") is reduced to as low a level as possible – recognizing that risk elimination is rarely possible when a process depends on the people actually performing the process. Furthermore, under such circumstances regular audits should be undertaken to verify compliance with specimen identity verification protocols.

For this reason several technological solutions using either bar codes or radio frequency identification (RFID) tags have been developed specifically for application in the IVF lab. Obviously neither can replace the need for at least two human-readable unique identifiers on any specimen container, since humans cannot read either bar codes or RFID tags, but they provide another level of specimen identity verification that is free from the risk of involuntary automaticity. Bar code-based solutions include *Matcher* (IMT International, Chester, UK; see www.imtinternational.com) and *Trusty* (Optimal IVF, Melbourne,

Australia; see www.optimalivf.com.au/html/trusty.html), while RFID-based solutions include *Witness* (Research Instruments, Falmouth, UK; see www.research-instruments.com/products/ri-elements/ri-witness; also Thornhill *et al.*, 2013) and *Lablogger* (Cryogatt, Buxted, UK; see www.cryogatt.com/).

Early concerns that the radio frequency electromagnetic radiation associated with reading RFID tags might be harmful to embryos were allayed by two-generation studies in mice subjected to 700 times the expected dosage of radio waves (see www.research-instruments.com/download/Mouse_Study_test_results_summary_for_export.pdf).

In addition to specimen identity verification, each of these systems allows for operator identity and time logging. *Witness* and *Matcher* also allow for full process mapping and enable checking that the correct specimen/container is being used at each particular step. *Trusty* is a simpler system in that while it verifies that each specimen/container belongs to the particular treatment cycle, it does not incorporate process mapping capability. Because of difficulties applying RFID technology at ultra-low temperatures, the *Witness* system cannot currently handle the cryogenic storage steps of cryobanking processes, although *Lablogger* is a specialized system with similar process control capabilities and is specialized for cryobanking. Being bar-code-based, both *Matcher* and *Trusty* can deal with specimens at both ambient and cryogenic temperature ranges.

As the value of such systems becomes more widely recognized, their implementation will spread. Currently many smaller labs think that such technology is only affordable by "big labs," which is highly debatable, especially when one considers that it is in smaller labs that the "lone worker" situation is more likely to arise, and hence where an electronic specimen verification system represents the only solution to operator-independent witnessing.

Protecting IVF laboratory staff from unfair litigation

As risk management moves from the manufacturing industry to healthcare there is a far greater – or at least more immediately obvious – impact of risk on customers' wellbeing. Although the underlying issue and driving force for risk management is patient safety, the increasing focus on financial risk, not just medical risk, has substantial implications for healthcare workers – and hence IVF centers.

A leader in the medical application of RCA stresses that "Errors must be accepted as evidence of systems flaws, not character flaws" (Leape, 1997). But even if the professions involved all agree that adverse events are the result of happenstance, multiple human errors that combine in a particular configuration by chance (Reason, 1994; Bogner, 1994), a situation with extremely negative emotional impact could arise if the unfortunate, and unintentional, victims obtained an RCA report describing the "causes" of their problem – and litigation could ensue. Because personal liability is a far greater risk in healthcare than in industry, issues of personal fear are correspondingly more prominent.

In addition, some organizations operate under a management culture of fear, which further compounds employees' worries and increases the likelihood of errors being concealed, cover-ups organized, and staff dishonesty in general. No center should instruct its staff to conceal errors, or to lie to patients under threat of dismissal or other punishment. Such behavior is unacceptable. In a decent, supportive work environment, where risk management and quality flourish, the following principles must guide all human resource activities (and be documented in all employees' contracts):

1. No-one will be punished for making a mistake;
2. Mistakes are always seen as opportunities for improvement;
3. If a mistake occurs it must be reported to the supervisor immediately and dealt with expeditiously;
4. Anyone who lies about a mistake or attempts to cover one up should be dismissed; and
5. All levels of management must adhere to and apply these same principles.

Protection of employees from personal liability is essential if any modern-thinking IVF center is to function without its staff living in permanent dread of litigation – a concern of everyone, not just clinical embryologists. To this end, centers must have fully detailed standard operating procedures (SOPs) documented and in place, complemented by comprehensive quality management and risk management programs. Then, so long as all staff members work within this framework, the center should have a legal (not just moral) obligation to indemnify its employees against personal responsibility for any adverse event that might occur, since it will have been a fault of the system. Naturally, in cases of mischief, dishonesty, or blatant malpractice the center's obligation would be nullified. Incompetence should also be the center's responsibility since staff selection and training are the employer's responsibilities, and staff members who cannot perform any of their duties should not be allowed to continue performing them. Systems for continuous employee appraisal, proficiency evaluation and competence testing should be implemented by the employer, with both participation and satisfactory performance being mandatory.

Conclusion

Although the great majority of IVF Labs (actually, IVF centers) probably do not have a formal risk management program in place, we hope that the material presented and discussed in this chapter will have provided sufficient insight to allow everyone not only to recognise the need for such activity, but also to make a start on developing risk management processes for themselves. Beyond the jargon and formalized processes of risk management lies another example of an area that is essentially common sense and which is readily amenable to the application of scientific method.

Chapter 10

How are we doing?: benchmarking

Benchmarking, basically, is the proof of what is possible. In a traditional business setting, benchmarking is the continuous process of measuring one's products or services against one's strongest competitors or those renowned as world leaders in the field. In its practical application for IVF centers, benchmarking can be viewed at three levels:

- Internal benchmarking: comparisons between centers within a group or network;
- Competitive benchmarking: comparisons against the direct competition; and
- Functional or generic benchmarking: comparisons against the "best-in-the-world" centers.

For an IVF laboratory, benchmarking can be seen as verifying that the laboratory outcomes and the center's clinical success rates are maintained, monitoring the implementation or amendment of processes to improve outcomes to match those of competing centers, and evaluating the development of better processes or technology to meet, or exceed, the performance of other centers. Benchmarking is the best way to avoid complacency.

There is also some confusion in how the term "benchmark" is used. For some a benchmark is a "minimum standard," while for others it is (more correctly) an "aspirational goal" defining what they wish to achieve:

Minimum performance values define criteria for basic competency: if you can't achieve at least this result then you shouldn't be doing it, should stop doing it, or should be stopped from doing it.

Aspirational goals define best practice, i.e. what you would like to achieve – although targets must always be realistic.

Clearly, for quality improvement purposes the latter sense is the important one, but the former can be used when troubleshooting or reviewing a lab for performance improvement opportunities.

The international society for clinical embryologists Alpha organized a consensus meeting in 2011 on defining KPIs and benchmarks for the cryopreservation of oocytes, zygotes, cleavage-stage embryos, and blastocysts by either slow freezing or vitrification methods. The report included definitions for the KPIs as well as consensus-based values for both minimum performance and aspirational goal benchmarks for each KPI (Alpha Scientists in Reproductive Medicine, 2012).

It is vital to remember that a benchmark relates to a process and a population of cases, not to the result of an individual patient's treatment. So if a process such as embryo utilization rate has a benchmark of 75%, then a case where only 40% of cleaved zygotes were suitable for transfer or cryopreservation on the day of transfer should not be automatically seen as "abnormal" or "a failure" – there can be many sound reasons for such an outcome (e.g. many post-mature oocytes at OPU). However, the proportion of cases that fall below the benchmark value might be another KPI to monitor.

Like systems analysis and process control (see Chapters 5 and 6), benchmarking requires the use of Indicators, things that are measured to determine how we are doing. But because benchmarking requires us to compare indicators between IVF labs or centers, it requires greater care in ensuring that these Indicators are calculated the same: we must not only compare apples with apples, but they must be the same sort of apples, e.g. Granny Smiths, and be ripe (i.e. "fit for purpose"). Such considerations are covered later in this chapter after we have established what sort of performance indicators we might want to use.

Sentinel indicators and adverse events

In addition to performance indicators readers will often find references in quality management texts to "sentinel indicators." Sentinel indicators are somewhat different to performance indicators, although the term is used with various meanings by different authorities. At its most extreme, a sentinel indicator is an unexpected occurrence involving death or serious physical or psychological injury, and is often qualified with the phrase "or the risk thereof" – in other words it is a marker of failure. However, in other areas of quality management a sentinel indicator can be anything that can be measured or quantified to monitor a process. Given this confusion we avoid the use of this term entirely.

Because of the nature of IVF we need both types of measurement: for success and of failures. Fortunately, most of the high-profile adverse events that can arise in ART are generally rare, although every occurrence is critical and anything less than complete correction is less than adequate, i.e. such an event would be seen as a system failure. However, many such accidents are in fact probably due to "the insidious concatenation of often relatively banal factors, hardly significant in themselves, but devastating in their combination" (Reason, 1994) – making them more-or-less unpredictable. What this means is that a whole lot of little things (quite probably individually not apparently of any major consequence) all manage to go wrong at the same time, and something dreadful ensues. So, if nothing else, effective risk management will help eliminate the occurrence of critical adverse events that do not fall into this extreme classification. But some of these "sentinel events" might be tolerable with certain prevalence, and it is the goal of risk management (essentially, quality improvement) to progressively reduce the frequency of such events, while accepting that some cannot be eliminated (which ergo cannot be defined as failure).

Therefore we need to use careful terminology to describe the different types of events. Critical adverse events can be termed just that, while measurements of laboratory processes (or any other operational processes within the IVF center) will not – hopefully – constitute critical adverse events; they are merely assessments that form the quantitative basis for quality control and quality assurance. Indeed, their existence is fundamental to the ability to monitor the results of any corrective action. To this end, such events can be termed "Indicators" ("KPIs" using ISO terminology) and confusion avoided.

KPIs are essential:

- For evaluating the introduction of a technique or process;
- As minimum standards for proficiency;
- For monitoring ongoing performance within a QMS (for both IQC and EQA purposes);
- For benchmarking; and
- For quality improvement.

How to choose Indicators

As already discussed, Indicators are crucial to the development, and maintenance, of a quality system. In accordance with the maxim "You can't control what you can't measure," the Indicators that are used should reflect the areas which, when controlled, will bring the most measurable benefit to the IVF program. So, for example, even though pregnancy rate is an important indicator of the overall program performance, it is not necessarily the most useful one in terms of benefit to the program's efficiency, finances, and operation. Nor is it especially useful for monitoring the operation of lab processes, since it is: (a) an endpoint that is well downstream of the lab, and (b) can be highly affected by non-laboratory (clinical and patient) factors.

It is quite likely that the most useful Indicators will differ from one IVF program to the next, since they will depend upon the areas being targeted for improvement. This is why accreditation authorities typically do not provide a list of "mandatory" Indicators beyond a few that reflect the overall performance of the clinic – it is expected that the areas of need will have been identified as part of each center's ongoing quality improvement process.

From the patients' perspective, apart from cost and location, a center's pregnancy rate and implantation rate are the most likely Indicators that will be sought. It is important, therefore, that everyone in the program understands that these rates are indicators of the center's performance as a whole, and not simply of the laboratory's performance. It is also important to realize that different IVF programs may have (indeed, will likely have) different definitions for their Indicators – therefore, it is essential that the definitions used for each Indicator are known before any attempt at benchmarking is made. Further discussion on the use of reference populations for reporting results as well as some general considerations of definitions of success rates and honesty in reporting pregnancy rates follows the next section.

Defining Key Performance Indicators (KPIs)

Any KPI must be defined fully and carefully:

- Define the process, biological or technical, that is to be monitored.
- Identify the specific endpoint of interest for that process.
- Identify relevant qualifiers (e.g. female partner's age).
- Identify confounders:
  - Biological factors, e.g. abnormal stimulation response and fertilization rate of oocytes;
  - Clinical practices, e.g. patient selection and fertilization failure;
  - Patient factors, e.g. source of sperm.

It is also essential that the definition of a KPI specify the exact data that are to be collected, as well as how they are used to derive the KPI value (calculation formulae, etc.).

A lab must then establish the appropriate periodicity for updating the KPI, e.g. monthly, each 30 cases, etc. But in small centers with low caseload it might take some time for a reasonable number of cases to be performed before an updated KPI value can be calculated. In this situation the KPI might be re-calculated using combined old and new data, e.g. 15 new cases and the last 15 cases used in the previous calculation. This will lead to some smoothing of the values, and concomitant loss of sensitivity, but at least an updated value will be available twice as often using such a "Tukey window" smoothing approach.

How many KPIs (or benchmarks) do we need?

This is a question we're often asked – and one to which there is no right answer. Any process that can be measured (which basically means every separate process) has, de facto, a KPI, and hence a benchmark (or both minimum standard and aspirational goal values) can be defined. And this works not just for the lab, but for any area of an ART center.

The following lists are only intended to be illustrative, to provide examples of the types of KPI that can be followed, under general sub-headings. Each IVF lab or center should establish their own set of KPIs that meet their specific needs from an operational perspective, in addition to others that are needed for external comparisons.

Program KPIs

- Pregnancy rates (should be broken down by female patient's age and procedure):
  - biochemical (positive β-hCG)
  - clinical (e.g. fetal sac or fetal heart at 7-week ultrasound)
  - ongoing (e.g. fetal heart at 7-week ultrasound or pregnancy).

- Implantation rates (should be broken down by female patient's age and procedure):
  - overall (e.g. [total number of fetal sacs seen at 7-week ultrasound]/[total number of embryos transferred to all patients in that age group and procedure type])
  - incidence of multiple implantation (e.g. proportion of pregnancies with >1 fetal sac at 7-week ultrasound).

Laboratory KPIs

Note that oocyte and embryo evaluations provide measures that are referred to as "grades": we strongly recommend not using the word "quality" as it can be very misleading, and be misunderstood by others.

- Oocyte grade and/or maturity (note: this is not actually a KPI of the laboratory's performance, but it does provide a description of the "source material").
- IVF fertilization rate (the proportion of inseminated oocytes which have 2PN the day after insemination).
- ICSI fertilization rate (the proportion of injected oocytes which have 2PN the day after injection).
- Poor or failed fertilization rate (e.g. the proportion of cycles in which <25% of inseminated oocytes fertilized).
- ICSI damage rate (the proportion of injected oocytes that degenerate during stripping, during microinjection, or immediately following the injection procedure, i.e. that are seen at the fertilization check).
- Zygote grade.
- Cleavage rate (e.g. the proportion of zygotes which cleave to become embryos).
- Embryo development rate (e.g. the proportion of cleaved embryos which are at the 4-cell stage 2 days after insemination; the proportion of cleaved embryos which are at the

8-cell stage three days after insemination; and/or the proportion of embryos which are at the blastocyst stage 5 days after insemination).

- Embryo fragmentation rate (e.g. the proportion of Day 3 embryos with <5% fragmentation).
- Embryo score or "grade" (e.g. the proportion of Day 3 embryos with the highest score).
- Embryo utilization rate (the proportion of cleaved embryos which were transferred or cryopreserved).
- Embryo cryosurvival rate.

Efficiency KPIs

- Number of tests handled by individual operators.
- Time lag between receipt of an enquiry and the response.
- Proportion of patient records which are complete.
- Number of telephone calls answered by a person, rather than by voicemail.
- Average delay between completion of a test and the publication of results.

Best practice KPIs

- Incident reports.
- Treatment complications.
- Infection and accident reports.
- Number of comments received per month (both positive and negative).

Laboratory operations KPIs

- Number of each type of procedure performed each week or month.
- Equipment malfunction reports.
- Equipment performance (e.g. amount of LN_2 required to top up a storage dewar; amount of CO_2 or pre-mixed gas used by each incubator; incubator temperatures).
- Rate of utilization of consumables (e.g. plasticware).

Financial KPIs

- Comparison of the service fees with those of other centers.
- Comparison of the cost of performing a procedure and the revenue it generates.
- Accounts payable and accounts receivable balances.
- Number of patient referrals per month.

When advising a lab on monitoring lab performance we recommend that they maintain a standard set of KPIs (with associated benchmark values) that allow them to be sure that each aspect of the treatment process can be monitored: basically this is the list of lab KPIs provided above. Additional KPIs might be employed from time-to-time when there is a particular need, e.g. when introducing a new procedure, or as part of a troubleshooting exercise. And obviously we also keep track of the program KPIs for monitoring overall performance.

Reference populations

Often there is a need to compare KPIs (usually some measures of clinical outcome such as pregnancy rates or live birth rates) across many IVF centers, especially for such purposes as a national registry. In these situations, each center's results are not just reported *en masse*, usually with stratification according to female patient age bands, but also in terms of some sort of "reference population" that is designed to be consistent between all the centers to allow direct comparison between the centers.

As an example of such a reference group, the following program KPI values were derived in 2002 for a lab that was running Oozoa lab systems, using cases where the women were <37 years, having their first IVF or ICSI cycle, and two 8-cell embryos were transferred per Day 3 ET:

- Pregnancy rate (67/105 cycles βhCG+ve) = 64%
- Clinical pregnancy rate (63/105 cycles had ≥1 sac at 7-week ultrasound) = 60%
- Ongoing pregnancy rate (58/105 cycles had ≥1 fetal heart at 7-week ultrasound) = 55%
- Implantation rate (88 sacs from 210 embryos) = 42%
- Multiple pregnancy rate (25/63 pregnancies were twins) = 40% (no triplet pregnancies).

We then used these values as benchmarks for labs that we were advising, and indeed still use them today for clinics that have not moved to primarily blastocyst transfers.

Obviously the more tightly the reference population is defined, the smaller it will be for any clinic. Hence for smaller IVF centers the dataset from which their reference population KPIs are calculated might be very small, and hence the actual results being used for comparison will have different degrees of statistical robustness. In this situation, confidence intervals are attached to the reference population KPIs so that their uncertainty of measurement can be stated and the KPIs compared meaningfully between all centers (e.g. as explained in the UK Human Fertilisation and Embryology Authority's information for patients; see http://www.hfea.gov.uk/fertility-clinics-success-rates.html).

A properly defined reference population must not only consider the demographics and etiology of the patients receiving treatment, but also technical aspects of the treatment modalities employed – especially the number of embryos replaced. A major concern related to so-called "league tables" of pregnancy rate per transfer was the possibility that some centers might transfer higher numbers of embryos to "compensate" for what were actually lower success rates per embryo transferred compared to other centers. In response to these concerns, both the SART and HFEA databases have now evolved to report the average number of embryos transferred per cycle, and the proportion of cycles using elective single embryo transfer. Ideally, the next step in the evolution of these and other databases will also include analyses of the implantation rate per embryo transferred.

The Canadian ART Register (CARTR) now includes the singleton pregnancy rate following elective single embryo transfer (eSET) in "optimal" cases, i.e. women <35 years having their first IVF or ICSI cycle and, although it is not specified, presumably Day 5 ET. In 2012, based on clinic-average results, the average value for this KPI was 49%, ranging between 27% and 74%, and the mean ±1 SD was 38 to 59, hence 59% could be taken as the aspirational goal benchmark. However, there are both benefits and limitations of using benchmarks derived in this way:

- Clinics within the group are able to compare themselves against the others.
- The "better" clinics within the group can be identified.

- Aspirational goal benchmarks can be derived based on what your competitors are achieving.
- But the benchmark value is pulled down by the "poor" clinics in the group.
- Comparing clinics within the group can be compared to others outside the group so long as the same reference group definition is used.

Applications of benchmarking

Internal benchmarking: This form of benchmarking considers comparisons between centers within a group or network. In Australia, the UK, USA, and Canada there are corporate IVF organizations who provide services at multiple sites, and for organizations such as these it is clearly important to be able to ensure that comparable performance and outcomes are achieved regardless of the location. However, ensuring comparability of KPIs will still depend on the achievement of operational standardization between the sites – a daunting task to say the least!

Competitive benchmarking: In the world of IVF, comparisons against the direct competition are an everyday occurrence. In the UK and the USA, the success rates of individual IVF centers are published – which patients then use in deciding which private unit to attend. Even when a national registry publishes center-specific but anonymous success rates, each center knows who they are, and the one with the highest rates will often "break cover" to try and gain commercial advantage.

Functional (generic) benchmarking: In a way, this is what centers are doing when they make decisions about what stimulation drugs or protocol to use, or which culture technology or products to use. Unfortunately, it is usually a completely invalid benchmarking exercise as there are very many more variables within the IVF process that need to be controlled than just the one under consideration. However, if an IVF center were to look to a world-leading program and attempt to replicate its operational systems as well as its technology, then comparisons against such "best-in-the-world" centers can be useful. Certainly when we undertake consultancy work in this area, we are employing generic benchmarking, since the technology that we have been involved in developing (e.g. Mortimer *et al.*, 2002a) has been successfully implemented – in conjunction with effective quality management systems – in many locations around the world with very comparable performance indicators.

Our current (2014) suggested benchmarks for cases where the women are under 38 years of age are:

Oocytes:	>85% MIIs and <5% GVs (at ICSI stripping)
Fertilization:	IVF: >70% of COCs inseminated are 2PNs at 17±1 h *p.i.* (effectively ~85% of the MIIs)
	ICSI: 70–75% of injected MIIs are 2PNs at 17±1 h *p.i.* (with <5% damage & degeneration rate)
Cleavage:	Early cleavage: >50% are 2-cells by 28±1 h post-IVF / 26±1 h post-ICSI
	>95% of 2PNs are ≥2-cells by 44±1 h *p.i.*
	>75% of 2PNs are 4-cells by 44±1 h *p.i.*
Embryos:	Day 2: >45% high grade 4-cell embryos at 44±1 h *p.i.*
	Day 3: >40% high grade 8-cell embryos at 68±1 h *p.i.*
	>50% of cycles with ≥2 top grade 8-cell embryos at 68±1 h *p.i.*

Utilization rate $\geq$60% at time of ET

Day 5: If routine Day 5 ETs, >60% zygotes to blastocysts by 116±2 h *p.i.*

Implantation: Day 3 ETs: 33 to 36%

Day 5 ETs: >45%.

Note that the assessment times used are in accordance with the Alpha and ESHRE Embryology SIG consensus values (Alpha and ESHRE Embryology SIG, 2011a,b).

Honesty in reporting results

As was intimated in the preceding section, clinical results and indicators can be manipulated quite extensively by altering the composition of the dataset. While the majority of IVF labs are probably honest, there are certainly many IVF centers, especially in highly competitive commercial environments, who are less scrupulous in their definition of KPIs. Perhaps fans of the BBC television series *Yes, Minister* and *Yes, Prime Minister* might consider this to be one of Humphrey Appleby's "irregular verbs"? *I employ properly defined reference populations to calculate my KPIs, your reference populations are subject to some bias, and he cheats on his success rates...*

This is not the forum for an extensive debate and analysis of honesty in reporting, but as scientists we should endeavor to define KPIs that will restrict opportunities for introducing bias or cheating, and that will facilitate communication and comparison between centers. Properly trained scientists are objective, and manipulation of research data or results constitutes academic/professional misconduct, and scientists caught doing this will suffer significant penalties from their institution and the journals in which they (attempted) to publish such results. Maintaining the same rigorous academic standards when reporting IVF success rates will benefit not only the patients but us as professionals.

Specifying systems

11

All the basic concepts and principles for the tasks that will be considered in this chapter have been covered in the preceding chapters. The purpose of this chapter is to provide particular examples of those concepts in practice, and to place the process of specifying the systems that will be used in the IVF lab in the "real world."

Regardless of whether we are choosing or specifying a technical procedure or a piece of equipment, we must consider it within the context of a process. General principles for specifying a system include:

- **What does it need to do?** This defines the technical specifications of the procedure or piece of equipment, as well as required or acceptable tolerances in its performance.

- **How well must it do it?** This relates to the performance as well as the reliability of the procedure or piece of equipment.

- **Will it last?** For equipment, what is the offered (or available) warranty and the availability, quality and cost of after-sales service and repairs.

- **Will help be available?** What support is available, either from the manufacturer of a piece of equipment or a reagent (e.g. culture medium), or from the originators of a particular technical procedure or method?

Selecting methods, devices, equipment, etc.

There are some simple rules to follow when selecting a method, piece of equipment, or a device.

1. Evidence-based considerations:
   a. Has the method, device or instrument been used by other IVF Labs?
   b. Are there established performance indicators for the method, device or instrument?
   c. How do the established performance indicators for the method, device or instrument compare to *your* internal benchmarks?

2. Regulatory approvals:
   a. Does the method, device, or instrument have necessary regulatory approval(s) from the authorities that govern your operations?
   b. Does the method, device, or instrument have any other regulatory approval(s) from other authorities, as indication of its quality and fitness-for-use?

Possible regulatory approvals include those from authorities such as the US Food and Drugs Administration, e.g. a 510(k) pre-market clearance, or CE marking within the European Union.

3. Follow the manufacturer's instructions:
   a. If the manufacturer has provided instructions on how to use the method (e.g. reagents or kits), device, or instrument, ensure that everyone is aware of them and follows them.
   b. If the manufacturer has provided instructions on how to store reagents, a kit, or a device, ensure that everyone is aware of them and follows them.
   c. If you have modified any of the manufacturer's instructions then ensure that your SOP describes the change(s) in detail. Maintain records of the development and validation studies that were performed to establish such changes in *your* lab.

4. Avoid known problems. If there are any known problems with the use of a method, reagent, kit, device, or instrument, ensure:
   a. that everyone is aware of them; and
   b. that your SOP includes all necessary details to ensure that they will not be repeated in your lab.

There are a number of issues, both general and specific, that have been established as significant sources of decreased outcomes in IVF lab procedures, and it is the responsibility of the lab director to be aware of what is in the literature and to either deal with the issue directly or, where it might be outside his/her jurisdiction or direct control, to bring any possible factors that might create adverse outcomes for the IVF center to the attention of the center's medical director. Failure to do so is not only unprofessional and unscientific, but could leave the lab director open to accusations of incompetence and perhaps legal liability. However, if a lab director were to bring such issues to the attention of those in charge of an IVF center and they decided, for whatever reason, not to accept – or to just ignore – the lab director's advice then those "executive managers" have assumed all responsibility for that decision, as well as any and all possible future liability.

While we do not recommend the routine use of such self-protection actions, there are some IVF centers where the lab has little or no say in such decisions but, nonetheless, is often blamed for anything that goes wrong. A written memorandum outlining the lab's scientific concerns, including references to the evidence upon which they are based, can save great acrimony – and possible future liability.

Can semen analysis be standardized?

It has long been recognized that assessments of sperm concentration, motility, and morphology can be subject to wide variations due to technical error. However, methods whereby this intra- and inter-observer variability can be reduced have been known for quite some time (e.g. Mortimer *et al.*, 1986, 1989; Mortimer, 1994; World Health Organization, 1999). The basic requirements are simple: (1) use robust methods; and (2) train the staff in the correct performance of the methods. The basic semen analysis courses run by the Andrology Special Interest Group of ESHRE, the European Society of Human Reproduction and Embryology, have provided eloquent evidence of the validity of this approach (Björndahl et al., 2002). Therefore the only reason that sperm assessments are not performed more reliably in many IVF centers can only be that the medical and scientific direction of those centers just doesn't care about sperm. This, of course, makes a self-fulfilling prophesy of the opinion that sperm counts, etc., don't have any value – how could observations with error components of up to 50% be taken seriously or used intelligently?

The relatively recent publication of the 5th edition of the WHO Lab Manual ("WHO5"; World Health Organization, 2010), and the related paper to substantiate the decision to decrease the reference value for sperm concentration from 20×10^6/ml to 15×10^6/ml (Cooper et al., 2010), caused some confusion in the male infertility field, but for little real improvement in patient management. Lars Björndahl's eloquent essay on the use and abuse of reference limits for the interpretation of semen analysis results (Björndahl, 2011) should be required reading for anyone performing or interpreting semen analyses. Unfortunately, WHO5 contains several significant methodological issues that many experts perceive to diminish the value of analyses performed according to that manual (see Barratt et al., 2011), and for that reason members of the ESHRE Andrology SIG's Education and EQC subcommittees prepared their own semen analysis handbook (Björndahl et al., 2010).

Reactive oxygen species and sperm preparation methods

It has been known since the late 1980s that the centrifugal pelletting of unselected ejaculated human spermatozoa can result in the generation of reactive oxygen species (ROS) within the pellet. These ROS can damage the spermatozoa to such an extent as to impair, or even destroy, their fertilizing ability (Aitken and Clarkson, 1988). A 1991 editorial raised an important risk management question: if a couple had an unsuccessful IVF cycle in which such iatrogenic sperm dysfunction may have occurred, and then had a successful IVF cycle in which a more appropriate sperm preparation technique was used, might they have grounds for legal action against the person(s) responsible for the earlier treatment attempt (Mortimer, 1991)? Subsequent research has confirmed the possible severity of this problem (Mortimer, 2000), and the issue, therefore, remains a valid concern.

Tomcat catheters

Although these catheters are sold as veterinary products, they were used extensively in the early days of assisted reproduction and are still used today in some IVF centers for intra-uterine insemination and even embryo transfer. In many jurisdictions their use for clinical applications is forbidden by the regulatory authorities, but not everywhere. Their attraction is their very low cost and reports that they perform as well as "proper" embryo transfer catheters (see Studies A and B in Table 11.1). However, not only have more recent randomized trials demonstrated Tomcat catheters to give worse clinical results (Studies E and F in Table 11.1), but both these trials were cancelled at interim data analysis due to the unacceptable prejudice the Tomcat gave to those patients. A report has described endometrial lesions caused by more rigid catheters, including the Tomcat (Marconi et al., 2003). Therefore, from an analysis of efficacy and safety, as well as considerations of regulatory approval, there would seem to be no place for the use of Tomcat catheters in a responsible IVF lab.

Table 11.1 Results of studies comparing the Tomcat and other catheters for embryo transfer.

Study	Pregnancy rate by catheter type					
	Tomcat[1]	TDT[2]	Frydman[2]	Wallace[3]	K-Soft[4]	Cook SIVF[4]
A. Gonen et al. (1991)	28%		16%			
B. Meriano et al. (2000)	47.0%	14.7%				
C. Wisanto et al. (1989)		9.2–19.4%	32.3%	19.2%		
D. van Weering et al. (2002)		20.5%			27.1%	
E. McDonald and Norman (2002)	20.5%					29.6%
F. Mortimer et al. (2002c)	28%					52%

Manufacturers:
[1] Kendall, Mansfield, MA, USA.
[2] Laboratoire CCD, Paris, France.
[3] Smiths Medical, Hythe, Kent, UK.
[4] Cook IVF, Eight Mile Plains, Qld, Australia.

Cryo buffers: the move from PBS to HEPES

In the mid-1990s, when Sydney IVF was eliminating patient serum from all its culture media, the serum component in the embryo freezing and thawing protocols was replaced by a solution of 45 mg/ml of HSA in normal saline (this being the albumin content of serum). However, in one lab the freezing solutions were based on a modified version of phosphate-buffered saline (PBS) that contained phenol red and it was noted that when straws were being seeded, the medium column had turned from the normal pink colour to bright yellow. Clearly there was a problem with pH buffering during cooling in the absence of serum, and this was confirmed by pH measurements. Advice from Dr John Critser led to the adoption of a TL-HEPES medium as the basal medium for embryo freezing and thawing in August 1996. Not only did the HEPES buffering allow for proper pH control during cooling, but the implantation rate per thawed embryo transferred went from 6.5% to 16.2% (Cullinan et al., 1998). Moreover, even when embryos that had been frozen in PBS-based solutions were thawed in TL-HEPES there was a significant improvement in implantation rate to 14.3%, indicating that the major damage was probably being done during thawing and washing to remove the cryoprotectant. Subsequently, a HEPES-buffered version of the cleavage medium (Mortimer et al., 2002b) was developed and has been used since that time (Cook IVF, 1999).

Research on the temperature stability of phosphate buffers has revealed that they are highly unstable at lower temperatures and therefore unsuitable for freezing and thawing media. Early success with embryo cryopreservation using PBS-based solutions was probably aided by the additional buffering capacity of the serum component, but with the replacement of serum by albumin it seems that embryo freezing and thawing solutions should not be based on PBS.

The mechanism for the adverse effect of the low extracellular pH remains unproven, but it has been shown that thawed hamster embryos are unable to regulate their intracellular pH for several hours, until proper homeostatic mechanisms are restored, and that this may be at least a partial explanation for their impaired oxidative metabolism and decreased developmental competence (Lane *et al.*, 2000).

A bit about engineering and temperature calibration

Calibrating temperatures

Because of the sensitivity of gametes and embryos to temperatures outside the physiological range, every IVF lab must do a lot of temperature measuring and checking to ensure that each piece of critical warming equipment is set correctly, and continues to function properly.

It is surprising that, even today, we still get told by proud embryologists or lab managers that all the workstations have been calibrated to 37.0°C. Unfortunately, it is not the heated surface that needs to be at 37.0°C but the gametes or embryos. This means that each piece of equipment combined with the specimen device needs to be calibrated to achieve this desired temperature. For example, when working in a K-Systems cabinet with a heated surface, the temperature of the surface should not be carefully set at 37.0°C, rather the temperature at the bottom of a "dummy" dish containing medium (or water), with oil if that's how it will be used, must be maintained at the target temperature – and the heated surface will, invariably, be slightly warmer. The magnitude of this differential will depend not just on what the dish contains but also its design, since the depth of the air gap that separates the base of the dish from the heated surface will adversely affect heat transfer, because it acts as an insulator. Moreover, different dishes have different size air gaps, from the small fraction of a millimetre for an ICSI dish to almost 2 mm for a NUNC four-well dish.

But the complexity does not stop here. If there is air flowing across the open dish then there will be an additional cooling effect that will be influenced by:

- The velocity of the air flow (since a faster flow will result in a larger mass of air per unit time flowing across the open dish);
- The temperature differential between the dish contents and the air (ΔT);
- The relative humidity (RH) of the air that is flowing across the dish;
- The surface area of the dish; and
- The presence of oil (which will prevent evaporation).

While the presence of an oil overlay will effectively eliminate the loss of heat due to evaporation (the latent heat of evaporation that is lost from the water as it evaporates), it will not influence the cooling effect due to air cooler than the specimen.

As a consequence of all the above factors, during "egg search" the follicular fluid is typically exposed to a constant stream of ambient temperature, low-RH air that induces constant evaporation of water from the dish, cooling the follicular fluid and also increasing its osmolarity. Clearly using a 90 mm or 100 mm diameter dish will exacerbate this cooling artefact compared to a 60 mm dish. Given the pervasive complexity of these cooling issues it should be quite apparent why we have chosen to work in controlled environment "IVF chamber"-type workstations since the early 1990s, and why the better-designed workstations achieve not just a negligible ΔT, but also a higher internal RH – as well as also permitting control of the pCO_2 of the circulating atmosphere inside them.

But returning to our Petri dish on a warmed surface model – which is still by far the most common modus operandi in IVF labs around the world. Taking the "egg search" model system, we obviously need to set the heated surface to a temperature that will allow the target temperature of 37°C to be maintained in the close vicinity of the oocytes (which should be in follicular fluid that has been maintained as close to 37°C as possible since its aspiration from the follicle, e.g. using a tube warmer) for at least as long as is required to complete the examination of the dish for oocytes. This means considering three temperatures and time:

T : the target temperature (37°C)

S : the surface temperature of the workstation

D : the temperature setting that is shown on the display of the controller (which should = S)

In practical terms:

1. Adjust the controller so that T is stable (as measured using a calibrated thermocouple probe);
2. Measure S (again using a calibrated thermocouple probe, ideally a surface probe); and
3. Note the reading D on the display.

Once the correct T has been verified then it will remain constant for that dish configuration so long as S is maintained. This means that on a regular (e.g. daily QC) basis, there is no need to re-verify T directly: so long as the configuration remains the same then T will be correct if S is correct. D is also noted in order to monitor that the relationship between the controller's display and the effective temperature achieved at the heated surface remains constant. If the relationship between D and S changes then the system needs to be re-calibrated – but only after the continued proper operation of the heating and controlling system has been checked, i.e. the heated surface device has been serviced and re-calibrated by a certified engineer using test instruments that have themselves been properly, and recently, calibrated.

The same approach must be taken for each workstation and each step in the IVF lab process, and other critical parameters also need to be verified by independent measurements, e.g. incubator CO_2, O_2, RH. In the andrology lab, reliable assessments of sperm motility, especially progression (since sperm velocity typically doubles between "ambient" temperatures of ca. 22°C and 37°C), require that heated microscope stages be used so that the slides (or other specialized chambers, e.g. Makler chamber) can be maintained at the physiological temperature of 37°C throughout the assessment.

Minimum daily QC for IVF lab equipment requires that the temperature control of each workstation is verified (by measuring S and reading D, and recording both values for posterity) at least once, usually before starting work each morning. That the system remains in control throughout the day is then assumed – and this is why real-time monitoring systems (e.g. Planer's *ReAssure* system) have such value, since they measure and log T every five minutes, entirely independently of the equipment's own controller, with zero effort by the embryologists (although D readings should be logged daily to monitor the constancy of the controller).

Of course, our independent measurements of T and S must be accurate, which means that each temperature measuring device used must be checked against a reference thermometer (which itself has been certified against an external reference device according to its manufacturer's specifications). This in-house calibration of thermometers or, more commonly nowadays, thermocouples, is very simple.

- Prepare a controlled temperature calibration system, e.g. a beaker of water at 37.0°C, where the 37.0°C is verified using a certified reference thermometer (TR).
- At the 37.0°C set point, determine the reading given by the thermocouple that is being calibrated (TC).
- Calculate the difference between the two values. Always calculate this as TR – TC so that if the thermocouple being calibrated is reading higher than the reference value the correction factor will be negative, and vice versa: if the thermocouple being calibrated is reading lower a positive difference value will be obtained.
- Write the correction factor, or "offset," on the thermocouple itself (e.g. write it on the connector), or at least have it readily available in a correction table that matches it to the specific thermocouple. Most thermocouples will be within ± 0.2°C, but this cannot be assumed.[3]
- Whenever a reading is taken using the thermocouple, add the correction factor to the reading before writing it down.
- Note: For the greatest accuracy, each thermocouple should be calibrated in conjunction with the particular meter (digital thermometer) with which it will always be used for making measurements.

If a thermocouple will be used across a wider range of temperatures then it should be calibrated across that range, e.g. for use between a refrigerator (*ca.* +4°C) and a water bath being used for heat inactivation of complement (*ca.* +60°C), then use a freezer compartment and a boiling water bath as the two calibration points. Hopefully the thermocouple will show a linear response across this range – this is exactly the same principle as performing a two- or three-point calibration of a pH probe (where the slope of the fitted straight line between the calibration points is usually referred to as the probe's "efficiency").

"Alert" or "alarm"? What does it mean when my incubator goes "beep"?

The typical immediate response is to ask "What's gone wrong?" But really understanding what a beeping noise means requires that you know the operational characteristics of the particular piece of equipment that is going "beep." Just because an incubator is beeping does not necessarily mean that there is a problem: equipment can go beep in order to communicate a variety of things, such as:

1. I'm operating normally, and have just reached the set-point – just like many kitchen ovens when they've finished pre-heating.
2. The temperature (or whatever is being measured) has exceeded the tolerance range. This is a warning or alert that the incubator's temperature is not within the expected range of the set-point (i.e. not within the control range), but not that it is malfunctioning or that a real problem has occurred (yet).
3. The temperature has exceeded its acceptable range, and might now cause harm to the embryos.

---

[3] As a good friend of ours has been heard to say many times: to assume makes an "ass" out of "u" and "me" . . .

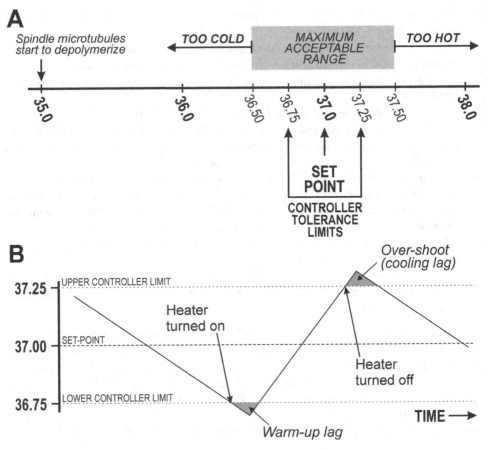

Figure 11.1 Temperature control.

Obviously situation #1 is perhaps more of a nuisance than a convenience; and, indeed, most incubators don't go beep to tell us this, they just stop flashing something on the display.

Situation #2, if it's not properly understood, can cause enormous frustration and problems – but no detriment to the embryos. Figure 11.1A shows how an engineer who is programming the firmware inside an incubator might apply temperature control limits:

Set-point: This is the desired operating value of the servo mechanism.

Controller tolerance range: This range is defined by upper and lower limits that are used to control the servo mechanism, these limits must obviously be within the safe operating range since the system cannot be allowed to exceed safe operating limits.

Acceptable operating range: This range is bounded by the limits that are defined by when the system is "out of control", i.e. "too hot" and "too cold": temperature limits beyond which oocytes or embryos can be damaged.

Situation #3 is obviously a problem, and one needs to know about it as soon as possible. Immediate action will likely be to move the embryos to another incubator while the problem is investigated and resolved.

Based on these definitions, the controller tolerance range limits can be seen as "alerts," warning you that the incubator is not within its pre-determined control range – but these are NOT "alarms," as the temperature is still within the acceptable operating range. Only if the temperature exceeds the acceptable operating range would a (different) beep denote a problem, i.e. giving an "alarm" that the specimens might be in danger. Obviously it is vital that "alerts" and "alarms" can be distinguished (e.g. different beeping sounds, or a flashing indicator light followed by beeping) – and it is essential that people in the lab understand the difference, both technically and in their biological significance. Imagine what would happen if a lab considered every "alert" to be an "alarm" and considered giving the patients a free cycle because their embryos were thought to have been compromised? No compromise has occurred when an "alert" is sounded: indeed, detrimental effects are only likely to have been suffered after experiencing an "alarm" state for a definable period of time, based on the actual temperature reached and the duration of the exposure.

The controller running an incubator's heating system operates according to the basic principles of a servo mechanism (see Figure 11.1B). The incubator is not being heated constantly, the heating system goes on and off according to some pre-determined limits. When heating is "on" the incubator warms to reach its set-point, and then the heater is turned off. The incubator then cools due to passive loss of heat until it reaches a lower control point, when the heating is turned on again. Clearly the lower control point must be above the temperature that is considered "too cold," especially since there can be a delay while the electrical current passing through the heating element actually starts heating it: but during this lag period the temperature inside the incubator must still remain above the critical "too cold" limit.

Clearly the tighter the control limits the better – but engineers must work within practical constraints and real world situations. Things that must be considered include:

- If the system only has limits defined by the acceptable operating range there will be substantial risks of exposing specimens to temperatures exceeding the "too hot" and "too cold" limits.
- If the control limits are set too tightly then "alerts" will be triggered too often, causing distress, stress, or just plain annoyance.
- If the control limits are set too wide then the risks of reaching, or exceeding, the acceptable operating range limits could be unacceptably high, e.g.:
  - If the heating system has significant inertia and the lower tolerance limit is set too low then continued cooling while the heater is warming up could lead to specimens reaching the "too cold" limit; or
  - If the heating system has significant inertia and the upper tolerance limit is set too high then continued heating as a result of a response lag could mean that the "too hot" limit is reached.

Traditional big-box incubators employed strategies to reduce their susceptibility to cooling within a room whose ambient temperature was typically 15–17°C lower. Insulation reduced the rate of heat loss, and water jackets increased the thermal mass of the incubator (as anyone who ever tried to move such an incubator without emptying it first would have discovered!), so there was more heat to lose.

Modern bench-top incubators do not have water jackets, and typically no insulation either. Consequently their control systems must be reliable, and operate within narrower control ranges. However, because their thermal mass is far less than the total mass of a big-box type incubator, their heating systems are far more responsive, allowing faster and tighter control of temperature. Good lab system design then requires that their electrical supply be protected – but this is no different to the real requirement for a big-box incubator – and, in fact, much easier to achieve since their power consumption ("draw") is far less, around 170 W for the Cook MINC and Planer BT37 bench-top incubators, compared to 500 W to 1000 W. There is therefore a much lower demand placed on the emergency generator and/or uninterruptible power supply (UPS) system (the latter often being used to maintain power while the generator starts up); and the Planer BT37 even incorporates a two-hour battery to carry it over the generator start-up period seamlessly.

The only downside of a bench-top incubator is its greater sensitivity to external cooling, e.g. drafts from air conditioning vents. Such cooling should not affect the incubation chambers due to their active heating of both bases and lids (unless the cooling effect is severe), but it can lead to condensation in the gas supply tubing within the gas humidification compartment, since that lid is typically unheated. Again, the Planer BT37 incorporates additional strategies to combat this sensitivity to environmental conditions: there is a large warm metal block with grooves (the "fish block") to hold the gas tubing and reduce its susceptibility to cooling, and also a perspex cover as a further insulator between the compartment lid and the fish block.

An extension of this understanding of a temperature control system is knowing why a simple water bath can only regulate itself at a temperature a certain distance from ambient temperature, typically something like 7°C above ambient. Because the heating elements are large, and remain hot after the heating current is turned off, they continue heating the water for a significant lag period. The water then cools slowly, losing heat to the environment, until it reaches a control temperature when the heating is re-activated – and the current then takes some time to warm up the heating elements. Given this "dampening" effect of the thermal mass of the water, the controller range needs to be quite wide. This is the reason why low-cost water baths can only be set to regulate at *ca.* 30°C or above. If more precise temperature control is required then a device must include not just a heating system, but also a cooling system, to reduce heating over-shoot (and the heating system would also counter cooling over-shoot); thereby achieving tighter control.

Practical examples

The following sections provide worked examples to illustrate the principles of specifying systems described at the beginning of this chapter. It is not the purpose of this book to provide specific recommendations of one technology over another, nor to recommend any one particular make or model of a particular piece of equipment. Rather, it is our goal to encourage readers to consider all relevant factors in making such decisions instead of simply continuing to do what they or their mentors have done before. Nonetheless, we have provided some comment on our preferences in light of the factors discussed. Although the following examples are not structured as formal FMEAs, those general principles clearly apply and interested readers should use the information presented here to construct FMEA tables (as described in Chapter 7) within the context of their own labs.

What sort of embryology workstation is best?

There are a wide range of possible configurations of microscope workstation where one can perform the various technical procedures involved in routine IVF. (This analysis does not relate equally to a workstation where embryos are processed for freezing and thawing since there are different requirements for temperature and pH control.) At the simplest level, the common modern alternatives include the following permutations:

Style of cabinet:
- Vertical laminar flow (VLF) cabinet
- Neonatal isolette-style "IVF Chamber"
- Class II cabinet

A horizontal laminar flow (HLF) cabinet has not been considered as it provides no protection for the operator.

Clearly, on the open bench is unacceptable since it provides no protection from contamination for either the oocytes/embryos or the operator.

Warmed stages: Everyone is aware that some sort of warm stage must be provided for microscopes where oocytes and embryos are being examined. The oocyte in particular is extremely sensitive to alterations in temperature: cooling causes the spindle to de-polymerize, risking aneuploidy of the resulting embryo if not all chromosomes re-attach to the spindle when it re-polymerizes as the oocyte re-warms to 37°C (Pickering *et al.*, 1990; Almeida and Bolton, 1995; Wang *et al.*, 2001). In addition, temperature shifts can affect trans-membrane transport and many intra-cellular metabolic processes. Consequently, human oocytes and embryos must be held as closely as possible to a stable 37°C. Furthermore, a significant, but poorly recognized, confounding aspect of temperature control during the microscopic observation of oocytes and embryos in dishes is that the design of all traditional disposable plastic dishes does not allow the base of the dish to come into direct contact with the microscope stage, so there is always an air gap (see Figure 11.2). Because air is a poor conductor of heat, this air gap greatly reduces the efficacy of heated stages, allowing the medium in dishes to cool below the temperature at which the heated surface is set.

Gassed enclosures: When working with bicarbonate-buffered culture media, a CO_2-enriched atmosphere is essential to maintain the pH of the medium. A study by Blake *et al.* (1999) revealed that not only do bicarbonate-buffered media take a long time to reach equilibrium, but they out-gas very much more quickly than previously assumed. For example, a Petri dish containing 5 ml of culture medium will out-gas after removal from a CO_2 incubator so that the pH has shifted above 7.45 within two minutes – and that after replacing the dish in the CO_2 incubator it will take 15 minutes to re-equilibrate the pH (see Figure 11.5, later). These differences are due to the relative magnitudes of the differential CO_2 contents between the equilibrated medium and air and between the incubator's atmosphere and the partially out-gassed medium. This study is discussed further in the later section on the use and need for culture oil.

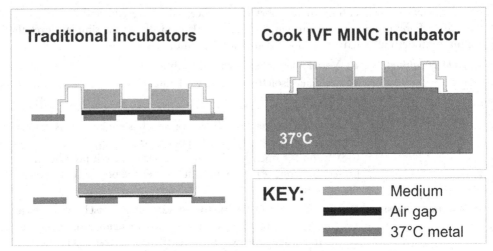

Figure 11.2 Diagram illustrating the existence of an air gap between traditional culture dishes and incubator shelves or warm stages and the lack of such an air gap in the Cook MINC mini-incubator. Because air is a poor conductor of heat, the temperature of the medium in dishes in the MINC incubator is re-established much more quickly.

In addition to standard commercial laminar flow and Class II cabinets there are also specialized workstation cabinets that are marketed for IVF applications, including the widely-used "K-Systems" cabinets which are either VLF or Class II cabinets fitted with warmed surfaces and gassing systems (K Systems, Birkerød, Denmark; www.k-systems.dk) and equivalent products from several other companies, including IVF Tech (Stenløse, Denmark; www.ivftech.dk), as well as the "IVF chamber"-type of controlled environment workstation, originally developed by modifying a neonatal isolette (Testart *et al.*, 1982). We have used this latter type of workstation exclusively since 1991: the original "IVF chamber" and more recently the "emCell-s" workstations from HD Scientific (Wetherill Park, NSW, Australia). While HD Scientific closed in 2013, the designer of these chambers, Dieter Regel, still services them from a company called Tek-Event (Round Corner, NSW, Australia; www. tekevent.com.au) and has just launched a third-generation workstation, the Cell-Tek chamber (www.tekevent.com/cell-tek/index.shtml).

The pros and cons of the principal alternative styles of workstation have been summarized in Table 11.2. Support for the contention that the IVF chamber-style workstation will provide better quality embryos and clinical outcomes remains limited (Mortimer *et al.*, 2001b), but several of the most successful IVF centers have chosen to use such workstations.

Choosing a CO_2 incubator

There are numerous factors that need to be considered when selecting a CO_2 incubator that go beyond the simple need for creating a CO_2-enriched environment for culturing gametes and embryos. Some aspects are technical, while others are more practical (see Table 11.3 for a description of these factors; also Figure 11.3).

Given the technical superiority of solid-state incubators using pre-mixed gas, we have been using these units exclusively since the late 1990s. Indeed, the project to develop the MINC 1000 incubator (Cook IVF, Eight Mile Plains, Qld, Australia) was initiated by us –

Table 11.2 Summary of the pros and cons concerning the principal alternative configurations for IVF workstations in relation to their ability to control extrinsic factors that can affect outcome.

Type of workstation		Temperature	Extrinsic Factor / Variable — CO_2 / pH	Air	Evaporation/Osmolarity	Rank
Vertical laminar flow cabinet	*Configuration*	Heated stage on microscope.	Sometimes a gas "funnel" is put over the dishes while they are *not* on the microscope, there is *no* protection while on the microscope.	Open to room air throughout unless gas funnel installed, in which case only exposed during observation.	Gas flowing into funnel or box is humidified by bubbling through a water bottle.	#4
	Effectiveness	Moderate. Still have air gap between bottom of dish and the heated surface.	Up to several minutes of exposure to room air during observation, also during holding if no gas funnel.	Exposed to VOCs and other contaminants in the room air at least during observation.	Moderate effectiveness while under gas funnel or inverted box, *no* protection during observation.	
	Ranking	4	=3	=3	=3	
K-Systems cabinet	*Configuration*	Heated stage built into the cabinet working surface.	Gas funnel usually installed for when dishes are *not* on the microscope, *no* protection while on the microscope.	Exposed to room air at least throughout the observation period.	Gas flowing into funnel is humidified by bubbling through a water bottle.	#3
	Effectiveness	Moderate. Still have air gap between bottom of dish and the heated surface.	Up to several minutes of exposure to room air during observation.	Exposed to VOCs and other contaminants in the room air at least during observation.	Moderate effectiveness while under gas funnel, *no* protection during observation.	
	Ranking	3	=3	=3	=3	
Older IVF Chambers	*Configuration*	Entire chamber warmed to 37°C.	Entire chamber has a CO_2-enriched atmosphere.	Air inlet has 0.22 μm filter, an in-line carbon filter can also be installed.	The atmosphere inside the chamber circulates continually over a humidification pan.	#2

Table 11.2 (cont.)

Type of workstation		Temperature	CO₂ / pH	Air	Evaporation/Osmolarity	Rank
				Extrinsic Factor / Variable		
	Effectiveness	All dishes inside the chamber are held close to 37°C whether on the microscope stage or not. Models with lower humidity can still have significant issues with evaporative cooling of open dishes.	All dishes are held under a CO_2-enriched atmosphere.	Exposure to room air minimized by semi-closed system	Humidity is maintained at "high" non-condensing levels, although the actual level achieved does vary with the model.	
	Ranking	2	=1	2	2	
Cell-Tek Chamber	*Configuration*	Entire chamber warmed to 37°C.	Entire chamber has a CO_2-enriched atmosphere.	Air inlet has 0.22 µm filter, an in-line carbon filter can also be installed. Air system is re-circulating with HEPA filtration and a photocatalytic system (Zander Scientific) to destroy VOCs.	The atmosphere inside the chamber circulates continually over a humidification pan.	#1
	Effectiveness	All dishes inside the chamber are held close to 37°C whether on the microscope stage or not.	All dishes are held under a CO_2-enriched atmosphere.	Equivalent air quality to a laminar flow or Class II cabinet plus VOC elimination capability.	Humidity is adjustable up to at least 70%.	
	Ranking	1	=1	1	1	

Table 11.3 Factors to be considered in choosing a CO_2 incubator.

General considerations	Factor	Comments
Practical	Capacity	• How much of the chamber will be available for use? e.g. Do you only place dishes at the front of the shelves? Do you use modular incubators inside the main incubator chamber? • How many cases will the incubator need to handle? Consider the number of dishes per case as well as the resultant frequency of door openings (a question of stability of the incubator's conditions). • What proportion of the lab's incubator capacity does each unit represent? If this is substantial then issues might arise during times when a unit is out of action, e.g. for cleaning or servicing.
Practical	Physical size	• Are there any space constraints in the lab? • Is there any problem with limited access for delivery of the incubator to your premises and getting it into the lab? • Will the new one fit where the old one was?
Practical	Ergonomics	• Will all your staff be equally able to access safely all shelves within the incubator? Besides the obvious issue of shorter embryologists not being able to reach the topmost shelves without using a step (which itself creates significant risk of injury and loss of embryos), will embryologists have to bend or kneel down to access the lower shelves of an incubator that is sitting on the floor? • Is the mains power switch liable to accidental operation? e.g. An incubator at floor level with the switch in the lower region of a side control panel could easily be knocked by someone using, for example, a floor cleaner.
Technical	Temperature control	• What are the tolerances of the incubator's operational performance around the "set point"? • How quickly does the incubator recover its temperature after a door opening? e.g. is a water jacket required for adequate performance? • How quickly do the contents of dishes placed in the incubator reach the desired temperature after being placed in the incubator (e.g. Cooke *et al.*, 2002; also Figure 11.1)?
Technical	CO_2 control	• Should you use an infra red (IR) or thermal conductivity (TC) based controller? Whereas historically TC controllers were cheaper and more reliable than IR units, improvements in technology have largely eliminated this consideration. However, the requirement for the temperature and humidity to be re-established inside the incubator chamber before a TC controller can commence re-establishing the CO_2 level makes them far less stable than units employing IR controllers (see Figure 11.2). • If the system has a built-in gas mixer (e.g. K-Systems G185 or the Embryoscope) then how is the composition

Table 11.3 (cont.)

General considerations	Factor	Comments
		verified? Not just internally, but also externally for independent validation. Also, how stable is this when the incubator has been opened? What is the recovery time?
Technical	O₂ control	• Do you want to use a low-oxygen atmosphere for embryo culture? It is well-established that a reduced pO_2 improves mammalian embryo culture *in vitro* (e.g. Tervit *et al.*, 1972; Bavister, 1995) and there is growing evidence that this also produces better-quality human embryos, especially if employing extended culture to the blastocyst stage (Catt and Henman, 2000). • If using a low O_2 system, should you use a tri-gas incubator or pre-mixed gas? • If using a tri-gas incubator, what will you use as the source of nitrogen (e.g. compressed nitrogen, liquid nitrogen vapor, etc.)? • If the system has a built-in gas mixer (e.g. K-Systems G185 or the Embryoscope) then how is the composition verified? Not just internally, but also externally for independent validation. Also, how stable is this when the incubator has been opened? What is the recovery time?
Technical	Air quality	• The quality of the air inside incubators has been raised as a possible source of concern (Cohen *et al.*, 1997; Mayer *et al.*, 1999), therefore steps should be taken to minimize the possible adverse impact of this factor on embryo culture. • If using traditional incubators then the quality of the air in the lab that will enter the incubators must be considered and appropriate steps taken to remove detrimental components such as VOCs. • If using an incubator or internal vessel that uses pre-mixed gas (e.g. modular incubator units or "bench-top" models such as the Planer BT37 or Cook MINC incubator), then that gas needs to be filtered to remove particulates and VOCs before entering the incubation chamber. This is an easier process to ensure than a system that allows room air to contribute to the culture atmosphere. Also remember that the capacity of a charcoal filter to absorb VOCs is greatly negatively impacted by humidity. • If the system has a built-in gas mixer (e.g. K-Systems G185 or the Embryoscope) then what is the impact of opening the incubator for specimen access on internal atmosphere composition? What is the recovery time?
Technical	Stability of the internal environment	• If the door will be opened more often than the recovery time for the incubator then should you buy a model with a split inner door? • For temperature stability do you need to have a model with a water jacket? While this was, historically, considered to be

Table 11.3 *(cont.)*

General considerations	Factor	Comments
		very important to ensure even heating of the chamber and for continued stability in case of power failure, this is far less important today due to improvements in incubator design and the expected availability of some form of emergency maintained power.
Safety	Power consumption and battery backup	• How much power does the incubator draw? When considering the provision of emergency maintained power this is a very important consideration, especially if the power is to be provided via a battery-based system. • If the incubator requires a lot of power then consider the total load that will be put on an emergency UPS or generator system. Bench-top incubators (e.g. Planer BT37 or Cook MINC) take much less power than do "big box" models. • Does the incubator have a built-in battery backup (e.g. Planer BT37)?

CO_2 recovery after 30 second door opening

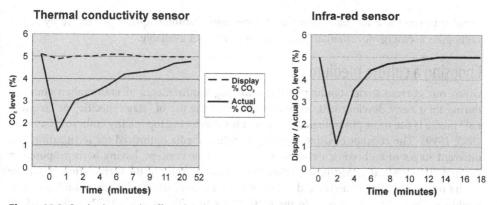

Figure 11.3 Graphs showing the effect of opening incubator doors on the CO_2 level and how its rate of recovery is affected by the type of CO_2 controller. The left-hand panel shows the results for a Forma Model 3360 incubator using a thermal conductivity type of CO_2 controller (data from the Forma Scientific website) while the right-hand panel shows the results for a Galaxy Model 170 incubator using an infrared CO_2 controller (data courtesy of RS Biotech, Irvine, Ayrshire, Scotland). Both incubators were fitted with a single inner door. Note the discrepancy between the actual CO_2 level and what was shown on the incubator display.

although we should state that because all development work was funded by Cook IVF we receive no financial rewards for their sales. The beneficial results of the value of these incubators (Mortimer *et al.*, 2002a) have been confirmed by other users in terms of both physical performance and clinical results (e.g. Cooke *et al.*, 2002; Mortimer *et al.*, 2002b; also Figure 11.4). One particular advantage of the bench-top of "solid-state" incubator is their much lower power requirement compared to traditional CO_2 incubators, making it

Implantation rates with Forma (•) and MINC (▪) incubators

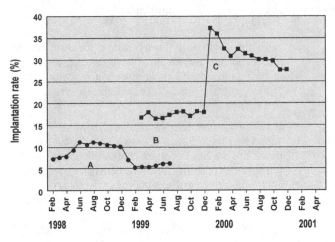

Figure 11.4 Graph showing the effect of incubators and culture media on implantation rate. Period A was using Forma incubators with a single-stage culture medium, while in Period B patients were allocated into either Forma (data points shown as circles) or Cook MINC (data points shown as squares) incubators, still using the same single-stage medium. Period C shows the further increase in implantation rate when sequential culture media were used in conjunction with the MINC incubators (the initial spike was due to January and February being quiet months in which pregnancy rate was affected disproportionately by small numbers of embryo transfers). Data generously provided by Simon Cooke, John Tyler, and Geoff Driscoll (then of IVF Australia – Western Sydney).

possible to run them for many hours on battery-based uninterruptible power supply (UPS) units even if emergency maintained mains power is not available.

Choosing a culture medium

Given our current understanding of the changing requirements of mammalian embryos during their early development, we still believe that the use of "stage specific" or "sequential" media is the most physiological approach for producing top quality embryos (Bavister, 1995; 1999). The concept of using a series of culture media optimized for fertilization and different stages of embryonic development is not a new concept, having been proposed in the mid-/late-1980s (e.g. Mortimer, 1986; Leese, 1990). Similarly, the formulation of culture media for mammalian gametes and embryos on the composition of oviduct fluid is a well-established concept, dating back to the early-1970s (e.g. Tervit *et al.*, 1972; Menezo, 1976; Quinn *et al.*, 1985; Mortimer, 1986). The subject of ART culture media is considered at great length in the recent book edited by Patrick Quinn (2014).

When choosing a culture medium to use in an IVF lab the following criteria are pertinent to making the best decision, not just from a scientific perspective, but considering important practical matters that are vital to the IVF lab's ability to provide a quality service.

Availability and stock:	The product not only needs to be available in your geographic area but ideally there should be a local agent or distributor who will hold some reserve stock in case of problems. While most culture medium companies require standing orders for regular supply, there must be a backup plan in case of a lost or damaged shipment – the IVF lab cannot be left without media under such circumstances.

Delivery and cold chain: The more stops along the way between the manufacturer and the IVF lab, the more difficult it is to guarantee the integrity of what is called the "cold chain," i.e. the knowledge that the media have been kept within their prescribed storage temperature range throughout the entire intervening period. If the product is manufactured in one country and then shipped to another via one or more intermediate places (e.g. the courier company's hubs of operation) then there must be a guarantee of how long it will take for this process to be completed, which must be within the ability of the packaging to maintain correct storage temperatures. Then, the agent or distributor must guarantee (and provide documented confirmation) that they maintained the proper storage conditions during their preparation of individual orders from their bulk delivery. Finally, the local delivery must be accomplished in a similarly expeditious manner to ensure that the proper storage conditions were maintained. Some companies ship temperature "tell-tales" or even loggers with their shipments, and it is up to the IVF lab director to decide how much documentation and confirmatory evidence (s)he requires to establish that the media were not compromised en route.

Cost: Obviously the cost is an important factor in selecting products for use in IVF, perhaps especially in countries where the fees paid for IVF are less than in more developed markets. For example, in India the cost of an IVF cycle is far less than in, say, the USA – yet labs in India have to pay substantially higher prices for their culture media than US labs due to higher freight costs plus customs duties and other taxes, as well as the costs of the local agents/distributors.

Suitability for use: Obviously IVF labs are going to choose culture media that have been established in the literature as suitable for human IVF and embryo culture. However, what is considered "best practice" changes over time as our knowledge increases. Very few IVF labs now prepare their own culture media, especially as the regulatory environment tightened and requirements for manufacture of these media according to GMP standards ("good manufacturing practice") became more widespread. There are also different regulatory requirements in different parts of the world (e.g. FDA 510(k) pre-market clearance in the USA, CE marking as a device in the European Union), and it is the responsibility of the IVF lab director to ensure that only properly registered media are used.

Quality control: A further dimension is the suitability of culture media for human IVF and embryo culture use, as defined by appropriate bioassays. All human IVF media manufacturers perform mouse embryo assay ("MEA") testing on their products and typically certify that they "pass" this test. But what does this mean? Here we must consider not only whether the MEA is "foolproof" in detecting all embryotoxic contaminants, but also just how reliable the MEA actually is. There have been situations in the past where media that passed the MEA with flying colors were later found to contain contaminants that, while not affecting the development of mouse embryos to the blastocyst stage, were certainly highly toxic to human oocytes or embryos *in vitro*. As for a comprehensive discussion on the reliability of the MEA, that could be the subject of another book on its own! However, the simple principles of quality management that govern the selection of products or services according to ISO 15189:2012 (see Chapter 6) require that the culture medium supplier not only provide documentary evidence that their product(s) "passed" whatever QC system they used (in this case the MEA), but that there is a statement of the uncertainty of those measurements. From basic statistical sampling theory, the fewer embryos used to performed the MEA the less robust will be the typical "pass" level of >80% blastocyst development.

Efficacy: While a particular culture medium product has been used by other IVF labs with a level of success acceptable to them, will its performance meet your expectations or requirements? Variations in other aspects of the culture system will likely change a product's ultimate performance, and hence careful comparisons of systems should be undertaken before deciding on a particular product or accepting a report of its efficacy. Cook IVF was the first IVF medium company to provide benchmark expectations of performance for its culture media products (Cook IVF, 1999), within the context of their complete culture system, based on the experience of the center that developed the products (Sydney IVF, under the scientific direction of one of the authors, DM). To the best of our knowledge, no other IVF medium manufacturer has yet followed this useful approach.

When/why do you need to use culture oil?

Why does an IVF lab use culture oil? What functions is it considered to perform – and what advantages is it perceived to confer or possible risks might its use incur? We have always been of the opinion that oil is a nuisance in the IVF lab and have restricted its use to only those situations where its benefits are proven. The logic for that position is considered briefly below – not in an attempt to "convert" other embryologists, but simply as the basic information upon which proper informed decisions can be made within the context of an FMEA, rather than a historical or "gut" opinion.

Prevents evaporation: Certainly a layer of oil over aqueous culture medium will greatly reduce evaporative loss of water from the medium. But how much of a problem is this? Obviously when working with microdroplet culture an oil overlay is essential to maintain the integrity of the droplets and prevent excessive evaporative loss. But what is the risk of evaporative loss to the extent that it causes an unacceptable shift in medium osmolarity for larger volumes of culture medium? With incubators whose internal atmosphere is properly humidified there is no serious risk of significant evaporative loss when using "open" culture in such vessels as Nunc plates or organ culture dishes (typical medium volumes = 0.5–0.8 ml).

Temperature stability: When questioned, many embryologists express the opinion that the use of an oil overlay will help maintain the temperature of the culture medium in the dish. When asked for the basis for that opinion, few are able to provide any source for the information, leading us to conclude that it is only dogma. Indeed, it has been shown that the presence of an oil overlay not only does not protect medium from cooling, but that the reverse effect is actually true (Cooke *et al.*, 2002).

Gassing and pH: Measuring pH in culture medium under normal conditions of use (i.e. an equilibrated system with a CO_2-enriched atmosphere) is extremely difficult, even using micro pH probes – which are notoriously difficult to use and keep calibrated. When developing the original "M91" series of culture media that were commercialized by Cook IVF as the Sydney IVF series of media (Mortimer *et al.*, 2002a) we did undertake some studies to verify that the pH of media inside the MINC incubators was stable within the desired range when the chamber was supplied with pre-mixed gas (6% CO_2/5% O_2/balance N_2). Having established that the media performed properly under correctly controlled conditions we concluded that there was no need to monitor the pH of media inside the incubators since it was determined only by the formulation of the medium, the temperature and the pCO_2 of the gas phase – all of which can be controlled independently. Clearly this is a simpler, more robust approach to quality control than attempting to make routine measurements of pH knowing that the proper measuring system is difficult to calibrate and very prone to fluctuation.

But what about outside the incubator, for example during fertilization checks or embryo assessments when the culture dish is exposed to room air? Or when culture dishes are placed in a traditional CO_2 incubator where the CO_2 level has been reduced by the opening of the door? Our solution to the first problem is to use IVF workstations with a controlled atmosphere, e.g. the IVF chamber (see above), but what happens when the control system is less robust? At the meeting of Alpha held in Copenhagen in 1999, Debbie Blake presented some studies on the dynamics of out-gassing of equilibrated culture medium either as drops under oil or as larger volumes in Petri dishes in a traditional CO_2 incubator (Blake *et al.*, 1999). Some of her results are shown in Figure 11.5, which clearly illustrates the following conclusions:

1. It takes longer to equilibrate 50 µl droplets of medium under oil than 5 ml of medium in an "open" dish.

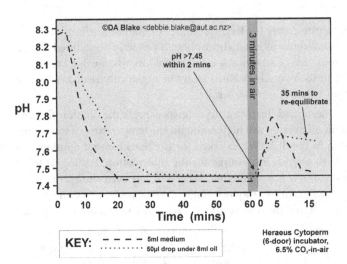

Figure 11.5 Graph showing the equilibration of either 50 μl drops of medium under oil (dotted line) or 5 ml of medium (broken line) in 60 mm diameter Falcon 3004 dishes. Dishes were then taken out of the incubator (a Heraeus Cytoperm fitted with a six-section inner door and running at 6.5% CO_2) and placed under an air atmosphere for three minutes before being replaced in the incubator. In both cases the pH of the medium had exceeded 7.45 within two minutes of exposure to air, and re-equilibration took about 15 minutes for the 5 ml of medium in a dish and 35 minutes for the 50 μl droplets. (Blake *et al.*, 1999; data generously provided by Debbie Blake).

2. In both cases the pH had exceeded the desired range (i.e. was >7.45) within two minutes of exposure to room air.
3. Re-equilibration after replacing the "out-gassed" dishes in the CO_2 incubator took about 15 minutes for 5 ml of medium, but about 35 minutes for the 50 μl droplets under oil.

In summary, it appears that not only does oil not slow out-gassing (i.e. it does not help protect against pH shifts), it actually hinders the re-equilibration of medium pH after exposure to room air. While further studies would be warranted to investigate this issue in more detail, in the meantime there would seem to be no benefit to using oil in terms of maintaining pH in culture media.

Time-lapse monitoring

Over the past few years, time-lapse monitoring ("TLM") of embryo development has evolved from a basic research approach to a technology that is available for routine use in IVF labs, in the form of the Embryoscope (Unisense Fertilitech A/S, Aarhus, Denmark; www.fertilitech.com) and Eeva (Auxogyn Inc, Menlo Park, CA, USA; www.auxogyn.com/eeva.php) systems. Leaving aside the current heated debate regarding the basis for some applications of this technology (Cohen, 2013) – this is clearly a very important research tool. In terms of improved clinical outcomes, however, at the time of writing the jury is still out, as there is still a dearth of published peer-reviewed evidence to support claims of improved outcomes using TLM. Indeed, there has only been one paper published that has shown an increase in clinical pregnancy rate in a study using the Embryoscope (Meseguer *et al.*, 2012): by 9% from 44.9% to 53.9%, equivalent to a relative increase of 20.1%. Unfortunately this study did not control for the incubator type, since the Embryoscope (a bench-top type of incubator) cases were compared to embryos cultured in traditional big-box incubators. Moreover, both systems used ambient pO_2, so a further improvement might be possible when low pO_2 is used in the

Embryoscope, since many labs have seen improvements in outcomes of similar or greater magnitude when simply converting from big-box incubators to bench-top incubators.

Hopefully more critical studies will be performed and published in the peer-reviewed literature very soon, as without them the conclusion of Kaser and Racowsky (2014) that "until such evidence accumulates, TLM should remain an experimental technology subject to institutional review and approval" cannot be revised.

Real-time monitoring systems for lab equipment

It is now generally accepted – if not actually a formal regulatory requirement – that IVF labs must have a system installed that will alert personnel when a piece of critical equipment (e.g. incubator or cryotank) malfunctions or fails outside normal working hours. Indeed, given the specific requirements for a QMS under the EUTCD's second technical directive (EU Commission 2006/86/EC), these compliance costs, especially those relating to the lab's clean room air-handling system, can constitute a major operating cost for a clinic. However, the means by which this essential element of the lab's quality management system is achieved can range from a simple dial-out alarm system that merely reports when an alarm condition is detected by the equipment itself, to automated real-time monitoring systems that not only make, and log, independent measurements on critical functions of equipment, but can also perform the same tasks for the laboratory's environment.

It is certainly true that a real-time automated monitoring system does have a significant up-front capital cost. But, rather than giving the "knee-jerk" response of declaring such a system "too expensive," each IVF lab should perform a comprehensive cost–benefit analysis of the ongoing costs of human-based monitoring and consider the total cost of monitoring the laboratory equipment and air quality over at least a three-year period. From the analysis of small, medium, and large model labs a clinic can expect to see overall savings from somewhere between late in the second year of operation for a medium lab, to mid-way through Year 3 for small and large labs (Mortimer and Di Berardino, 2008). Given the worldwide shortage of trained clinical embryologists, this should make automated monitoring systems both financially and operationally attractive from a management perspective. Automated real-time monitoring systems also exemplify the fundamental management principle of the well-run modern IVF lab: "work smarter, not harder."

Choosing an ART database

Ideally every ART center needs to have a comprehensive specialized ART database system that will manage all medical record information, allow management of treatment cycles in real time (including all laboratory processes), and enable queries and reports to be derived from the data. To aid centers in considering their information systems strategy we have prepared a summary of what we believe are reasonable current expectations for a serious ART database.

Essential functionality:

- Must accommodate same sex couples (including two males), single women, and surrogacy, including allowing partners or donors to change from one treatment cycle to the next.

- Must accommodate all forms of treatment, e.g. IUI and donor insemination cycles, not just for IVF/ICSI cycles.
- Must accommodate diagnostic andrology data: full semen analysis, antisperm antibodies, trial washes, sperm DNA fragmentation testing, computer-aided sperm analysis (CASA) of sperm movement characteristics (kinematics), sperm function tests, etc.
- Must include donor gamete (and embryo) sources, as well as those third-parties' screening and matching information.
- Must include appropriate data entry fields for working with sperm from all possible sources (including surgically retrieved).
- Must include endocrine tests as well as any other lab test results on either partner (and donors).
- Demographics information must be linked between the lab, clinical, and admin sections of the system (so it can be maintained by admin staff rather than lab staff).
- Scheduling module must include lab procedures and diagnostic testing (e.g. semen collection rooms).
- Scheduling module must generate task lists for lab procedures and diagnostic testing (also for other areas, including nursing, clinical, and admin).
- Must allow for entry of complete data, not just summary data, at the level of individual eggs and embryos. This includes element scores for multiparametric grading systems.
- Must allow for more than one observation of oocytes or embryos per day, as well as issues such as re-insemination (or repeat fertilization check after rescue ICSI).
- Must be able to store digital images/video clips for each oocyte/embryo at each observation point from OPU through to ET, including pre-/post-biopsy and pre-/post-cryopreservation.
- All grading schemes must be user-definable.
- Must accommodate lot numbers and expiry dates for all contact materials at the level of individual oocytes and embryos (to facilitate sibling oocyte/embryo studies, etc.). Ideally this should be via "templates" so that a group of products can be changed together, e.g. to facilitate media trials.
- Operator ID must be recorded for every process step. There must be an audit trail, including date and time stamps, for all data entries/changes.
- Deleted information from a record remains in the database and can be viewed/retrieved for audit purposes.
- Witness ID (human or electronic) must be recorded for every process step.
- Cryobank module must be linked to the procedures, so a cryobank location can be assigned from the specimen data entry screen, and vice versa for when using cryopreserved materials. This must include being able to see all empty cryotank locations when making assignment decisions.
- The cryobank module must integrate with billing for ongoing cryostorage.
- All procedures or tests must include provision for coding and prices for integration with billing.
- Clinical notes templates (e.g. for patient calls by embryologists) must be modifiable without great investment of time and effort.

- Completion of data submissions to national registry (or registries). Should also include the ability to generate a "missing data" report to facilitate completion of data collection prior to data compilation and submission.
- The system needs to include an "alerts" feature (e.g. medical for latex or penicillin allergies, financial for unpaid accounts, etc.) that can warn users of a patient's status when entering data or viewing results.

Essential reports and statistics:

- Full semen analysis reporting.
- Lab summary reports for treatment cycles.
- Outcome reports (including for cases with +ve β-hCG results, fetal sac, fetal heart, live birth).
- Lab KPIs (for QC and QA).
- Staff proficiency reports, e.g. ICSI damage rates.
- Activity/workload reports.

Highly desirable functionality:

- Capability for paperless operation, including all data entry "live" in the labs.
- Image capture capability should include andrology, so as to capture images/videos of unusual samples.
- Contact materials should be controlled based on lot number and expiry date, including warnings if an attempt is made to use an expired product.
- Test and procedure scheduling should allow for workload projection to facilitate staffing requirements, media ordering, etc.
- Interfaces to main instrumentation: endocrine analyzer, CASA machine, ultrasound machines.
- Ability to interface with external pathology lab test requisition and results systems.
- Ability to operate via, and control, user-definable processes. Should include each process step, and essential issues such as patient ID verification, witnessing, and confirmation of consent.
- Should maintain lists of patients being followed-up, e.g. 7-week pregnancy scans, birth data.
- Shewhart charts for KPIs.
- Activity/workload reports can be broken down by staff member.
- Prospective and retrospective analysis of planned events.

"Imminent" functionality:

- Touch screen data entry, especially for lab data.
- Ability to enter data, especially within the labs, using tablets via wi-fi.
- Ability to generate "intelligent" reports, i.e. where the report comments are based on the data fields.
- Ability to assign a "lab plan" to a case, i.e. a template that includes pre-configured process steps and appropriately configured data entry screens for the intended treatment. Also needs to allow for changes to the intended treatment modality, e.g. IVF conversion to ICSI, Day 3 ET to Day 5 ET, and perhaps IUI to IVF conversion.

- Display of task lists for an area (e.g. diagnostic lab, IVF lab, and other clinic areas) on a large monitor in the area. Staff can then see waiting tasks and "pick" their tasks (ideally should also include control of required staff competency, with provision for supervised training).
- Witnessing function should be able to be interfaced to a third-party system, e.g. *Witness* or *Matcher*.

Creating a quality IVF lab

Creating a quality IVF lab is neither simple nor a short task. Certainly it is easier to create such a lab when one is starting afresh with a new facility, but most IVF labs don't have that opportunity, they have to re-build and re-organize what they have – usually while having to maintain services with already limited human resources. Nonetheless, it is a daunting task that many lab directors will have to face anywhere that accreditation is pursued, but especially within the European Union in implementing a quality management system in accordance with the requirements of the EUTCD.

There is no single "right" way of doing this, no cookbook recipe that can be followed to achieve this goal. Each IVF lab will have to develop their own strategic plan in response to their unique combination of circumstances. However, the general principles described in the earlier chapters of this book will provide the background and framework for doing this, and the techniques and approaches we have described will provide a basic tool kit. But an open mind combined with comprehensive multidisciplinary knowledge is a vital pre-requisite for success.

In the final chapters of this book we will try and create a "road map" to reach this goal. But first we need to consider some aspects of managing the IVF lab's most precious resource, its people.

12 Human resources: finding (and keeping) the right staff

"Teamwork" is a huge buzzword in modern business, with the ability to create and/or assemble a winning team considered to be one of the hallmarks of leadership. For a team to function well, there must be mutual trust, respect, and cooperation – what Simon Sinek refers to as the "circle of safety" (Sinek, 2014). While each member of a strong, successful team has the knowledge, skills, and confidence to be a "star" in their own right, they also understand that this talent is shared by all the members of the team – and they each have the generosity of spirit to allow everyone to shine. It is precisely because each person in a winning team is a "star" that they are sought after by competitors who are hoping to create their own winning team. It is then incumbent upon the manager of a winning team to ensure that the effort and success of everyone in the team is recognized and rewarded – otherwise the team might be lost.

It is the same for the IVF center, and for the IVF lab, since a strong, functioning team is probably the greatest key to success. Recruitment and retention of good embryologists is a challenge. However, it is a challenge which must be met, because if you don't respect and look after your people, you have a fundamental flaw in your approach to quality. This is also a fundamental failing for accreditation.

In this chapter, we will discuss the types of people you need to look for when developing your team, and some of the strategies for holding onto the team once it is established and successful. While the examples are related to embryologists, many of the concepts are relevant to everybody who works in the IVF center.

Who makes a good embryologist?

Of course, to have a strong team, you need to have good people. But how do you know who to hire? It is quite possible that good embryologists are born, not made. We have found over the years that some of the best embryologists were hired as trainees on the basis of their personality traits, rather than their formal qualifications. Of course, an embryologist must also have a good background in reproductive biology – a degree in biological sciences is a reasonable requirement – but this should be the *first* step in the selection of staff, not the *only* one.

In essence, a good clinical embryologist will have most or all of these traits:

- Natural leader
- Well-developed sense of responsibility and accountability
- Able to work independently
- Self-starter
- Works well in a team
- Enjoys a challenge

- Perfectionist
- Strongly empathic
- Goal-oriented
- Energetic
- Honest
- Intelligent
- Creative.

It is also important to ensure that each person hired has the ability to meet the requirements of their job description. All applicants for a position must see the job description for that position as part of the interview process, and all of the requirements should be discussed fully.

Training: the importance of teaching "why" not just "how"

After you have found the right people for your team, they need to be trained, or re-trained. There must be a formal orientation and training program, with a comprehensive review process to ensure that training is adequate. However, because you are trying to build a team composed of creative individuals, there is always a risk that even trained people will think of a "creative" way to do a task, ignoring the SOP. As we have already discussed in Chapter 6, this is a very dangerous tendency, and one which will adversely affect the IVF center's quality management system.

The best way to stop this potential drift away from the SOP is to ensure that each person in the team understands why a particular procedure is done in a particular way. This is illustrated in the story of a young woman who moved away from home and had to cook on her own for the first time. Her flatmate noticed that whenever she was going to roast a piece of meat, she always cut off a corner of the raw meat, and asked her why she did that. The answer was "That's how my mother always did it, and she's a really good cook." Eventually, this habit drove the flatmate crazy, so the girl called her mother and asked why she cut off a corner of the meat before she roasted it. The answer was "I only have a small roasting pan, so if the piece is too big, the fat would drip into the oven, so I always cut off any part that doesn't fit into the pan to keep the oven clean." Clearly, the "why" asked a bit earlier would have helped the household budget!

In the lab, the best approach is to give the "why" as part of the "how." In other words, the rationale for a particular procedure should always be explained at the same time the procedure is being taught. This is helpful in ensuring that the SOP is respected, and it is also a good way to illustrate how all the processes in the lab are inter-related, and how they are each related to physiology. This should be sufficient to emphasize the importance of not deviating from the SOP, since, as a living document, it is the result of many years of experience. Furthermore, understanding the procedural and physiological bases for a procedure are necessary in troubleshooting, in developing improvements in methods, and in formulating research questions – each of which are skills required in a good clinical embryologist.

Competency-based accreditation and certification

Once a trainee is comfortable with the "why," it is then time to focus more fully on the "how" and facilitate their achievement of competency in each task. The concept of competency in training of embryologists and other laboratory professionals is becoming more widespread, in association with national certification and accreditation requirements. An international survey of these requirements was reviewed and discussed at the third international consensus meeting hosted by Alpha, held in Antalya, Turkey in May 2014.

For example, in Canada, the achievement of competency in a range of laboratory techniques and skills is a pre-requisite for certification as a Laboratory Professional by the Canadian Fertility and Andrology Society (CFAS). Their philosophy for a competency-based approach to training and evaluation is to promote the professional role of ART laboratory staff (www.cfas.ca). The CFAS expects that an ART laboratory professional would have the following competencies:

- Safe work practices
- Obtaining and processing of gametes and embryos
- Communication
- Quality and risk management
- Critical thinking.

In addition to these competencies, a lab supervisor or director must also be competent in:

- Communicating effectively
- Ethics and integrity
- Inspiring a shared vision and enabling laboratory personnel to act
- Critical thinking (further aspects)
- Facilitating organizational change/improvement
- Developing others
- Resource management
- Building teamwork and collaborative partnership
- Achieving results
- Self-confidence, self-control, and personal motivation.

Staff appraisal

As in all quality systems, there is a need to measure the effectiveness of staff performance. This is managed through the much-maligned staff appraisal process, which often causes stress and distress to staff and managers alike. However, it is possible to perform the staff appraisal in a constructive, non-threatening manner that both provides a record of progress and achievement and identifies areas of staff interest and opportunities for professional development. Our appraisal tool is designed to be completed by the staff member before the meeting, so that the meeting can be used as an opportunity to discuss the issues raised. The areas covered by the appraisal include:

- Self-assessment of performance, based on contributions and initiation of quality activities, and on customer focus;
- Evaluation of areas of weakness and strength, both personally and of the IVF center;
- Personal goals, both immediate and short-term;
- Identification of additional training needs;
- Verification of the completeness of the current job description; and
- Demonstration of understanding of responsibilities under occupational health and safety and infection control legislation.

By documenting this information in the annual appraisal tool, it is possible to maintain a record of each staff member's progress and affirmation of adherence to the relevant legislative requirements, as the staff member must sign their own appraisal to demonstrate that the information given is complete and correct. This is helpful in the day-to-day management of the clinic, and also in demonstrating compliance with requirements to verify that staff are aware of their obligations under occupational health and safety regulations, as well as with the IVF center's safety policies and manual. In addition to this, many accreditation schemes also include expectations that management will regularly seek input from all staff members on issues such as educational needs, as well as suggestions for improvements to the fabric of the IVF center and its general functioning.

The key to the success of the process is not to wait until the annual review time to communicate with staff about how they are doing. If someone is doing well, then this should be acknowledged at the time. More importantly, if someone is not doing well, this must be addressed urgently – there is more at stake than worrying about feeling awkward, since the success of the clinic is heavily influenced by the success of the laboratory systems. That way, once the annual appraisal rolls around, there shouldn't be any surprises, which opens the door to a constructive conversation reviewing the past year and planning for the next.

Why other people should be trying to steal your staff (and why they will be unsuccessful)

If you have managed to assemble and/or create a winning team, then, by definition, they will each have the knowledge, skills, experience, and confidence to be a star in their own right. It is a great compliment to you as a team leader or manager if your stars are being actively recruited by other clinics. However, since your staff are your greatest asset, you don't want make a present of them to your competitors. The way you get people to stay with you is to:

1. Ensure that they understand their value to the team;
2. Ensure that their contributions are recognized, illustrating that the team values each of its members; and
3. Create opportunities for them to "grow."

Frustration as a result of inadequate recognition is a significant problem in a team environment like IVF, and it is one of the major reasons that people will move themselves and their family across a city, a country, or the world just to work in another IVF center.

Different types of rewards

The size of a person's salary is a concrete demonstration of their value, and is a reward for many years of effort. It seems logical, then, that if a person is receiving a high salary, they will be satisfied enough to stay working for you. However, the higher a person's salary, the less motivating money becomes, and some people are motivated by factors unrelated to money. If their needs are not satisfied, or at least recognized, these people will find somewhere more amenable to work.

To keep employees' interest and motivation (and therefore to maintain a healthy and productive lab), there must be a consideration of:

- Internal motivation – personal belief in, and commitment to, the work; and
- External motivation – rewards, recognition, and personal growth.

Internal motivation is achieved when employees have a strong personal belief in the company's goals and processes. In the case of an IVF center, the contribution the lab team makes to patients' lives can be a very strong motivational factor. Ensuring that the lab staff have contact with patients, perhaps as cursorily as introducing themselves to couples before procedures, is a way of ensuring that the importance of their role is continually reinforced. Self-confidence is another major factor for internal motivation. When a person feels that they are performing an important role in the best possible manner, their self-satisfaction is itself a reward. In the same way, if someone does not have internal motivation, then they can never become a good embryologist.

External motivation comes from rewards given in formal recognition of a job well done. The most obvious reward is salary, but it can also be:

- More vacation days
- Flexible work hours to allow for family commitments
- More office space
- An enhanced health plan
- Increased contributions to a retirement plan
- Personal health programs, e.g. quit smoking classes, or gym membership
- Professional development, e.g. in-house education, support for formal qualifications
- Development of research projects
- Time for formal presentation of research results (i.e. writing papers)
- Support to attend conferences (and associated travel opportunities).

Because each person's needs are different, there should be a policy supporting two-way communication about the rewards program. To ensure staff morale is not damaged by rewards being offered indiscriminately, they should be given only as formal recognition of a job well done. Poor performance should never be rewarded, and there must also be a policy for effective discipline and punishment. It is also important that all staff be treated fairly, with rewards and/or discipline related strictly to work performance.

It should be understood that external motivation is not going to make someone with poor, or no, internal motivation into a good worker. Its value is in helping to ensure that a good worker maintains their internal motivation, and so will be less likely to look somewhere else for recognition and satisfaction.

Development of a career path

In addition to the rewards discussed above, creative, energetic, intelligent, goal-oriented people (like successful embryologists) also need to have long-term goals, such as a career path.

In almost every organization, the normal structure of the organizational chart is that of a pyramid (Figure 12.1). However, in an IVF lab there are – or one hopes to have – more senior embryologists than junior ones, yet there is only one lab manager or lab director (Figure 12.2). So how can a lab director provide a framework for professional development within the necessarily restrictive career structure of clinical embryology? One tactic that has worked well is to identify areas of specialized interest or responsibility within the laboratory that can be awarded to those senior embryologists who are motivated to seek them

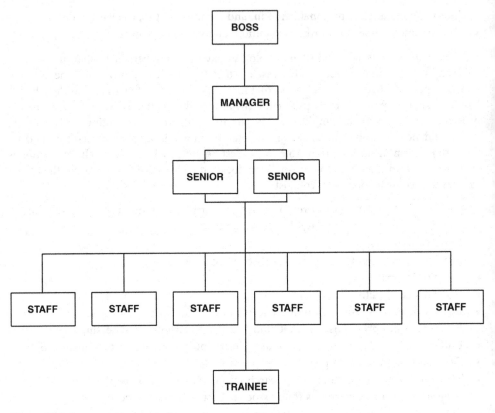

Figure 12.1 An organization chart of a generic company hierarchy.

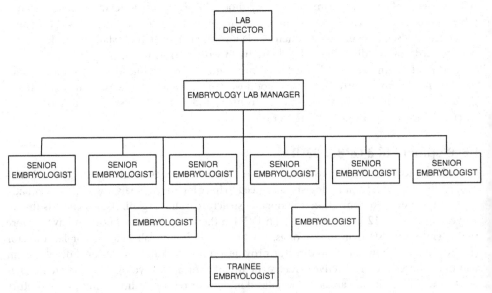

Figure 12.2 An organization chart showing the ideal situation for an IVF laboratory.

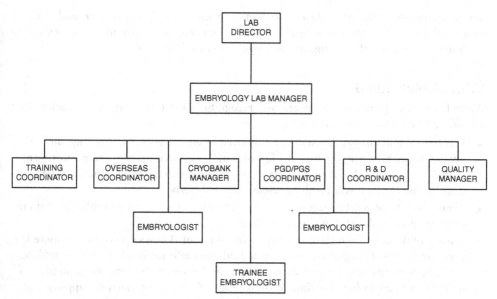

Figure 12.3: An organization chart for an "ideal" IVF laboratory showing how the assignment of "special responsibilities" can help create a career structure for the senior embryologists.

(Figure 12.3). Rewards can then be provided after they have demonstrated achievement in the extra role.

Delegation

Delegation, if done well, can be another very useful tool in developing and motivating employees. From the manager's point of view, it frees up time needed for other projects. From the delegate's point of view, it is a tangible expression of the manager's trust and confidence in their abilities. It is also an opportunity for the delegate to demonstrate talents which may not be needed in their day-to-day work (e.g. graphic design skills in making a poster). However, if the wrong person is delegated to do a task, or if the ground rules are not laid out in advance, it can be a disaster. For delegation to be successful:

- The right delegate must be selected – this is the same as when hiring someone, i.e. their skills must match the job description;
- The reason and goals for the task must be explained clearly;
- There must be a strict deadline given for the presentation of the completed project; and
- Once the task is delegated, there must be *no interference* from the manager – the trust given in the delegation of the task must be respected.

Another benefit of judicious delegation is that it gives the manager the opportunity to observe the delegate's approach to completing the project, which is a very useful way to test someone's ability in a new, expanded role, *before* taking the step of promoting them to it. This is crucial to ensure not only that the person could be happy with a new role, before proposing it to them, but also that they are capable of fulfilling the role. In this way, one can prevent the promotion of someone into a role which is too difficult for them – thereby avoiding the "Peter Principle" (after Laurence Johnston Peter (1919–1990)), i.e. "employees within an organization will advance to their highest level of competence and then be promoted to and remain at a level at which they are incompetent" (The American Heritage® Dictionary of the English Language: Fourth Edition, 2000).

Other considerations

Apart from these principles of reward and recognition, there are some other factors that should be taken into consideration:

- It is critical that enough lab staff are employed to ensure adequate coverage on the busiest days, and sufficient time off for all staff. It is unreasonable, and a short-term solution at best, to rely on people being good-natured enough to sacrifice their personal time for the clinic; it will result in resentment and burnout.
- There needs to be good communication to ensure that any looming problems within the team are dealt with promptly and effectively.
- Space and time are important – in an environment of "knowledge workers," there is a need for creative thought, and this is achieved most effectively when there is sufficient time and workspace. It is not reasonable to expect someone to generate good ideas if they are not able to find the time to think, and if they are not given the appropriate inputs – such as access to journals – and a supportive environment.

The humanitarian workplace: positive approaches to stress mitigation

The provision of ART offers a wide range of potential stressors, and it is important to recognize this and to develop strategies to mitigate the impact of stress on everyone in the clinic. These stressors can range from poor leadership through to the assimilation of change, and personal performance expectations. While it is critical that everyone work their hardest to provide a quality service to patients, it is also critical that the act of doing this work should not cause emotional damage, as this affects quality of life, as well as quality of service. The "humanitarian workplace" acknowledges the importance of both of these qualities, and strives to provide an environment that nurtures both.

Leadership

No matter how great the "raw material" is in terms of the staff members on the team, the team will fail in the absence of effective leadership. There is a huge amount of information available about leadership, but it was summarized most effectively by Harry Gordon Selfridge: "The boss drives people; the leader coaches them. The boss depends on authority; the leader on goodwill. The boss inspires fear; the leader inspires enthusiasm. The boss says "I"; the leader says "WE". The boss fixes the blame for the breakdown; the leader fixes the breakdown. The boss says "GO"; the leader says "LET'S GO!""

Great leaders have a strong belief in themselves, and in what they are doing. They understand their goals and they are totally on board with their aims. In this case, that means that a great leader, and a great team member, will believe completely in the importance of offering the best ART service to their clients/patients (since the "client" might be another member of the clinic, referring doctors, or service providers). Being fully invested in the belief is critical to ensuring success – as Simon Sinek states "People don't buy *what* you do, they buy *why* you do it" (Sinek, 2009). In other words, it doesn't matter if you have the smartest-looking, shiniest clinic in the world if you can't back that up with the fundamental commitment to quality and service in all areas.

There is no value to be realized by driving people – it is much more effective to encourage people to be the best they can be, to be their coach. This means that it is important to focus on the objective at all times – which is to give the person you are coaching the tools and opportunity to be the best that they can be. This can be a frustrating exercise, especially when the person you are coaching has not yet mastered the skill they are learning. But then, if you look at parenting as the ultimate type of coaching, it is obvious that the coach has to allow mistakes to be made as a form of learning – so long as the mistakes are made in a controlled environment, and their effects can be isolated or at least contained. Effective leadership also includes a mentoring role. It should be the aim of everyone who is responsible for a team that they can be replaced in the case of an emergency, or just as part of the progression of life. Ideally, there should be no thought of a mentor being threatened by the success of their mentee – in fact, the success of the mentee is a tribute to the mentor, and of benefit to all. If the mentorship process highlights shortcomings in the mentor's skills, then instead of being a threat, this is an opportunity for improvement – and, perhaps, an opportunity for the mentee to gain some teaching experience. Having the confidence to allow this type of role reversal requires a high level of mutual trust and respect, and is another example of the benefit of developing a "circle of safety" within the team(s).

While it is standard to think of leaders as being the most important person on the team, and therefore that their needs should come first, this isn't the most effective way to ensure success. In fact, the leader of the team should provide service to the team as a whole – ensuring that everything that is needed by the team to function properly is available when (or better still, before) it is needed. It's as though whenever anyone in the team is engrossed in what they are doing, say looking down a microscope, and reaches out a hand to grab the next thing they need, the leader has made sure that whatever it is will be there and ready to be used. In this way, the leader is like the master and the servant to everyone on the team – providing direction and motivation, as well as the means to achieve the goals.

This is also true for information management, in terms of communication between the team and the rest of the clinic, including clinic management. The lab director needs to function as a "bilateral semi-permeable membrane" – ensuring a two-way flow of useful and constructive information, while filtering out the "static."

Effective leadership also requires fiscal responsibility against a background of ensuring best practice. It is vital to be up-to-date with the newest technology and approaches, but there needs to be a critical evaluation of the likelihood of any advances leading to improvements in your system. It isn't logical to assume that adopting a new technique or incorporating a new technology into your lab will result in the same percentage improvement in outcomes as reported from other labs. If your lab is already performing well in relation to the benchmarks you have set, then you first need to consider how the innovation could be incorporated into your systems, and how it could solve a problem that you are experiencing. In the case of disruptive technologies, like ICSI, this is a fairly simple cost–benefit analysis. ICSI offered the possibility of genetic parenthood to couples for whom this had previously been out of the question, so the benefit to patients was obvious and it was worth the investment in equipment and training to be able to provide the service. However, this is not so obvious in the case of more incremental advances, and so the investment and

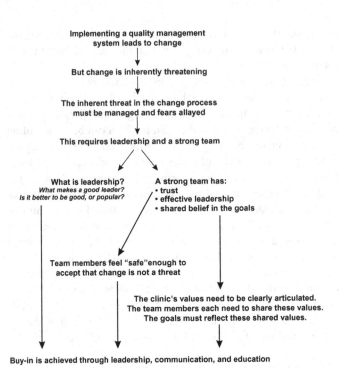

Figure 12.4 Factors in change management.

Implementing a quality management system leads to change

But change is inherently threatening

The inherent threat in the change process must be managed and fears allayed

This requires leadership and a strong team

What is leadership?
What makes a good leader?
Is it better to be good, or popular?

A strong team has:
• trust
• effective leadership
• shared belief in the goals

Team members feel "safe" enough to accept that change is not a threat

The clinic's values need to be clearly articulated. The team members each need to share these values. The goals must reflect these shared values.

Buy-in is achieved through leadership, communication, and education

potential disruption to service during the training period must be weighed against the magnitude of the likely improvement.

Managing change

The implication of the quality improvement cycle is that change is always possible, and even likely (Figure 12.4). As humans, we are inherently resistant to change, and so expecting everyone to embrace something that we are conditioned to avoid sets up a potential conflict within everyone in the lab, and even across the clinic.

Change for its own sake can be a very destructive force. Change is always disruptive, and if seemingly random changes are simply imposed upon people then the changes are almost certain to fail (unless they make people's tasks simpler). The rationale behind the decision to change systems and processes has to be made clear to everyone involved, to encourage their buy-in. In planning any type of change, the relevant processes and systems need to be considered to identify which areas of the clinic and which people in particular will be involved. The purpose of this is not just to ensure that introducing an "improvement" in one area doesn't cause a potentially catastrophic problem in another area, but also to encourage communication between all areas of the IVF center and to break down silos.

Managing change is a difficult process. There will always be fear and concern on the part of the people most affected by the change. For example, when bench-top embryo culture incubators were first being introduced, a number of embryologists felt that they would be deleterious to embryo development, and acting (as they believed) in the best interests of the embryos, they refused to use them. This fear was based on a "feeling," rather than on any evidence, and time has shown that this "feeling" was incorrect. Sometimes, it just isn't possible to convince someone that improvements are just that – rather than threats. This means that change needs to be planned in an inclusive process – by ensuring that everyone involved can appreciate the rationale for the change, and has input into developing the solution and planning how the change will be implemented.

Change from the management perspective

Change usually comes as a result of lots of protracted meetings at the management level, where the need for change and the relative value of the alternatives is discussed and debated at length. Finally, the best option is agreed upon and a decision is made to go ahead. It is often not until the next step, that of implementing the change, that everyone at the staff level hears for the first time that something is going on. This can result in frustration on both sides, as management has already gone through the whole process of deciding whether change is necessary, and then mapping out what needs to be done – so doesn't see the need to "waste time" going over it all in detail again; while staff feel that change has been imposed by the "higher-ups" without reference to the minutiae of the day-to-day running of the company. Unless management can identify and deal with this potential disconnect, meaningful change will be difficult to achieve.

Change from the staff perspective

From this perspective, change is something to be feared and resented. This fear often manifests itself in pushback and brings up trust issues, often expressed through questions and comments such as:

Fear

- Am I doing something wrong?
- Aren't I good enough?
- Will I be able to perform in the new way?
- How will I gain competency?
- Is it going to be harder/more complicated?
- Will I lose face if I have to ask for help?
- Will I be made redundant?
- Will I be judged?

Pushback

- There's no point in making a change
- It will be too hard
- It's dangerous
- It's unproven and patients and/or outcomes will suffer
- It will take me longer and I'm already too busy

Trust issues

- The boss doesn't understand what we do or what the change will mean
- They haven't thought it through
- They're just doing it to save money
- Nobody cares what we think.

If these issues are left unaddressed, this leads to a feeling of disenfranchisement amongst the staff, which in turn leads to resentment and a loss of commitment ("if they don't care about me, why should I care about them?").

In introducing and managing change, it is critical to work through these issues to sell the change concept:

1. Be honest with yourself about why the change is needed – is it solely for economic reasons, or are there other reasons as well? Make sure that there is a solid rationale for the change – otherwise there will be a *lot* of upheaval just for the sake of change, which is not an effective expenditure of time and energy (and staff goodwill).
2. Ensure that the change respects the clinic's core values. Ideally, these should match your core values – since it is very difficult to work in an environment that is at odds with your values.
3. Distill the explanation of the need for change, conveying the "why" before the "what."
4. Discuss this openly, and with everyone at once – and be prepared to listen and to heed everyone's concerns and comments. Work to allay fears in exactly the same way as you would perform a risk assessment – for each concern, identify whether the proposed change will create the perceived problem, and assess the likelihood and potential magnitude of the problem.

Overall, the key to managing a successful and productive change in practice is open communication, along with honesty and respect on all sides.

Mindfulness

We have noticed that often the very traits that make someone a good clinical embryologist can also hold them back in their career. The ability to continually evaluate situations and project the range of outcomes is critical in making judgments about embryo quality, which is directly related to the likelihood of pregnancy, and becomes second nature. Unfortunately, this can then spill over into other areas of life, with the result that people can become very judgmental, and then hypercritical, not only of themselves but also of others. This inevitably leads to increased levels of stress, as it seems that nobody is able to live up to the impossibly high standards that are being set. Sustained high levels of stress are the cause of a wide range of physical, emotional, and behavioral problems, which together lead to burnout and poor health, while significantly increasing the risk of errors along the way. In caring for staff, and providing a healthy and supportive workplace, it is therefore critical that the potential for stress be acknowledged, and strategies developed to assist people in managing their stress levels.

One approach in reducing work-related stress is "mindfulness." Mindfulness, which has its roots in Buddhist beliefs, is basically the practice of being non-judgmentally aware of your own body, emotions, and thoughts – in other words, observing without analyzing. Training in mind-based stress reduction (MBSR), as developed by Jon Kabat-Zinn, has been gaining significant attention over the past decade or so, and there has been a corresponding exponential increase in the number of papers published about mindfulness – from an average of 3 per month in 2005 to 57 per month so far in 2014 (based on a PubMed search of "mindfulness"). Some of the most recent studies have reported significant reductions in stress in healthcare professionals, with concomitant improvements in the quality of patient care (Regehr *et al.*, 2014; Asuero *et al.*, 2014). There is also evidence that the practice of mindfulness can promote neurological changes, suggesting a physical basis for the observed improvement in psychological wellbeing (Singleton *et al.*, 2014).

While it would certainly be impractical to suggest that everyone in the lab spend all their time in meditation, it is possible to apply the concepts of mindfulness as part of the work day. Being able to focus on the task at hand is critical to confidence and success. So the first step should be to clear the mind of distractions – such as analyzing why the last case wasn't perfect, or thinking about everything else that needs to be done in the day, etc., etc. Achieving this can be as simple as first deciding what to do next, and then before you start getting set up for that task, pausing to take five deep breaths while letting go of all of your thoughts and focusing totally on your breathing. As simple as that sounds, the act of focusing on those breaths gives the mind the opportunity to reset and get you ready to start on the next thing.

Does any of this really matter?

One of the most common responses to the question of investing time and energy in human resources is that there really isn't that much value in it, since it doesn't affect the outcome for patients. But having a positive workplace, with staff who are invested in their work, benefits everyone, including the patients. Indeed, there is now a whole field of study related to the effect of toxic behaviors on productivity. For example, in a 2009 study of the impact of incivility on performance, Christine Porath and Christine Pearson surveyed several thousand managers and workers in a range of American companies, and found that among those who reported being on the receiving end of rude behavior:

- "48% decreased their work effort
- 47% decreased their time at work
- 38% decreased their work quality
- 66% said their performance declined
- 80% lost work time worrying about the incident
- 63% lost time avoiding the offender
- 78% said that commitment to the organization declined."

Clearly, a non-supportive work environment can have far-reaching effects on the success of the business.

We recently heard of a clinic in which the laboratory had been rendered a toxic workplace by the previous lab director, with the result that the lab staff were traumatized about going to work, and had basically given up, only doing the minimum necessary to get through the day before they could escape. The new lab director spent the first few months working to improve the morale of everyone in the lab, re-building their confidence and treating them with care and respect. Since everyone was still threatened by the concept of change, and hence highly resistant to it, there was no attempt to modify any of the laboratory systems during this time. However, as people became more invested in their work, there was an improvement in outcomes, and after three months, the pregnancy rate had increased by 50%. This is a great example of how quality pays, and it will be interesting to see how much further their success rates are improved when it is possible to introduce improvements in the lab processes.

The end of the road

Letting someone go can be a truly heartbreaking experience, particularly when the "fit" just isn't right. However, when people's fundamental values don't align, then no amount of negotiating, counselling, or coaching will make it better. Hopefully, in such a case this disconnect will have already been noticed and discussed as part of the performance appraisal process, and so the need to end the work relationship will not come as a shock to the employee. Alternatively, if the person has wilfully violated company policy, for example by lying or stealing, then the termination needs to be managed swiftly. In all cases, attention should be paid to the safety of the person being fired, as well as to the safety and integrity of the clinic and the clinic team.

Finally, it should be remembered that no matter how great the team, how good the "fit," and how supportive the work environment, people *will* leave. Hopefully, their decision will be due to personal circumstances rather than to dissatisfaction. Therefore, as a quality initiative, it is important that exit interviews are carried out, to determine *why* the person is leaving, in case areas for improvement can be identified. For example, this is the opportunity to ask what the person would change about the organization (assuming anything was possible). It is also the opportunity to ensure that the person knows that their value is recognized, by asking the hypothetical question of whether they would consider coming back again in the future.

Illustrative example of a well-controlled laboratory

There are many ways of running an IVF Lab, and in this chapter we provide an illustrative example of a well-controlled lab. It is by no means the only way in which a lab can be organized and operated, and it is certainly not necessarily perfect from every lab director's perspective. In this "concept lab" we have integrated organizational, technical, and technological systems to create a lab in which one can be reasonably confident not only that the equipment is properly calibrated, but also that it continues to operate within expected parameters, and that procedural (including specimen custody) risks have been minimized. The overview considers a typical "fresh" IVF process from the laboratory perspective, commencing with oocyte retrieval (OPU) and culminating in embryo transfer (ET). Issues upstream of oocyte retrieval, such as stimulation and triggering – which will effectively determine the competence of the primary incoming "raw material" (the oocytes), and which will largely pre-determine the outcome of the entire process – are clinical aspects that are the responsibility of the medical director.

The material has been structured into four sections:

1. Environment (conditions inside the lab/procedure-room clean room)
2. Contact materials (culture media, tubes, dishes, etc.)
3. Equipment
4. Lab processes.

Details for each individual step, item, or aspect, include a description – a brief summary of the relevant SOP(s) – and a list of the specific control mechanisms for that item, with evidence to verify control or reveal uncertainty. For the purpose of this exercise, the laboratory is taken to be one that employs the authors' current general operational recommendations: environment-controlled IVF workstations (Cell-Tek Chamber, Tek-Event, Round Corner, NSW, Australia); Cook KFTH tube warmer (Cook Medical, Bloomington, IN, USA); Planer BT37 bench-top incubators (Planer/Origio) supplied by pre-mixed gas at 6.0% CO_2/5.0% O_2/balance N_2; the Cook Sydney IVF culture medium suite (Cook Medical) in conjunction with PureSperm density gradients and NidOil culture oil (Nidacon, Göteborg, Sweden); IVF Witness (Research Instruments, Falmouth, UK); and the ReAssure real-time monitoring system (Planer, Sunbury, UK). Tubes and culture dishes are from SparMed, BD Falcon or Nunc. All observations and other data are stored in the IDEAS database (Mellowood Medical, Toronto, ON, Canada).

Environment

Air quality

Description: The clean room suite is served by a primarily re-circulating HVAC system (maximum 15% fresh air per pass) that provides at least ISO Class 7 HEPA-filtered air into these rooms.

- The system includes Zandair PCOC3™ photocatalytic units that remove VOCs and also effectively destroy airborne microorganisms (including bacteria, viruses, and fungal spores).

Control mechanisms:

- The HVAC system is certified at commissioning by a specialist company and re-certified on an annual basis.
- The lab has test equipment for measuring particulates, VOCs, and ideally a specialized formaldehyde testing device. These units need to be re-calibrated regularly by the manufacturer or specialized biomedical engineer.
- Formaldehyde should be undetectable.

Laboratory ambient temperature

Description: Temperature control within the clean room suite is achieved via the HVAC system. The temperature is designed to be comfortable for the lab staff; temperature control and protection of gametes and embryos is achieved through the various systems and equipment described in this overview.

Control mechanisms:

- The thermostat is located in an appropriate place, away from undue solar heating effects.
- Independent temperature sensors are installed in each laboratory and connected to the ReAssure system.
- Display values from the local displays on the ReAssure system sensors are logged at the start of each day by the duty andrologist or embryologist.
- Separate independent verification of temperature is also performed periodically using a hand-held digital thermometer that has been calibrated in-house against a certified reference thermometer.

Real-time equipment monitoring system (e.g. Planer ReAssure system)

Description: This system monitors a series of temperature (T°C), %CO_2, humidity (%RH), and event or status sensors to monitor the following pieces of critical equipment at 5-min intervals:

Embryology workstation:	T°C, %CO_2, and %RH
Medium (CO_2-in-air) incubator:	T°C, %CO_2, and %RH
Culture (Planer BT37) incubators:	T°C (the incubator's internal data logging capability is also linked to the system)
Andrology (air) incubator:	T°C
Microscope heated stages:	T°C
Fridge-freezers:	T°C and door open status
Cryostorage dewars:	T°C and LN_2 level

Lab gases supply: Low pressure status for each gas

Room temperature: $T°C$ and %RH in each laboratory

Control mechanisms:

- Critical out-of-range parameters trigger audible alarms to lab staff on a 24/7 basis, and call-out alarms to cell phones outside lab operating hours.
- The lab manager can access the system for either real-time or historical data, generate graphs from within the system, and export data to Excel.
- The lab has independent devices for measuring temperature (including a certified reference thermometer) and percentage CO_2 to verify any questionable values, and to provide ongoing confirmation of operation of the ReAssure system's sensors.
- In case of any issues, or for system updates, Planer engineers can access the system from the UK via the internet.
- The ReAssure system server has UPS power as well as being on the emergency generator power panel.

Contact materials
Culture media

Description: The primary components of the system are fertilization, cleavage, and blastocyst media (all bicarbonate-buffered, requiring a CO_2-enriched atmosphere to maintain the correct pH_e), and gamete buffer (HEPES-buffered for use under an air atmosphere).

- Culture media must be shipped and stored at +2 to +8°C.
- Culture media have an approximately 4-week usable life from time of receipt under correct storage conditions.
- Once opened a bottle is not used for more than 5 days.
- Media are not used for culture for more than 48 hours following prior overnight equilibration.

Control mechanisms:

- Media are ordered on a fortnightly basis.
- Upon arrival, the internal temperature of the shipment container is verified as being between +2 to +8°C. If this is not the case then the shipment is rejected.
- Culture media are stored at +4°C to +8°C in a refrigerator that is monitored by the ReAssure system.
- Expiry dates are controlled and the lot/batch number of each medium used for every lab event is recorded on the lab forms and in the database.
- Bicarbonate-buffered media are equilibrated overnight prior to use in a CO_2 incubator (bench-top or CO_2-in-air incubator).
- In the event of an untoward culture finding the lab supervisor immediately considers what has happened to contemporaneous cases that are within the lab system.
- Any pattern of lot/batch usage that might coincide with untoward culture findings is reviewed by the lab supervisor/manager.

- If there is any occasion to even suspect that a batch of medium might be related to an untoward culture finding, the lab manager and/or laboratory or scientific director can contact other users of the Cook media system nationally and internationally to enquire whether any other lab(s) might be having similar experiences.

PureSperm

Description: PureSperm discontinuous density gradients are prepared by diluting the stock 100% PureSperm product with Gamete Buffer to avoid pH shifts when held under an air atmosphere.

- Unopened stock PureSperm is stored at ambient temperature, and at +2°C to +8°C after opening/aliquoting (aliquot flasks are dated). Under these conditions the shelf life of the product remains unaffected from the date set by the manufacturer.
- 40% and 80% (v/v) colloid dilutions are prepared in batches and aliquoted into ready-use quantities that are stored in the refrigerator.

Control mechanisms:

- Batches of the 40% and 80% (v/v) colloid dilutions are identified by the preparation date, and used within 10 days.
- The ReAssure system logs can confirm maintenance of appropriate storage conditions.
- At the end of each afternoon the requisite number of "gradient kits" is placed in an air incubator to warm to 37°C ready for use the following morning.
- Gamete Buffer is dealt with as described above.
- Expiry dates are controlled, and the lot/batch number of each stock product used recorded on the lab sperm preparation form and in the IDEAS database.

Culture oil

Description:
- When oocytes or embryos are cultured in microdrops (typically 20–50 µl) the drops are covered by culture oil to prevent evaporation of the medium that would result in deleterious changes in medium osmolarity.
- Microdrop techniques are typically used only for ICSI and extended/blastocyst culture (i.e. from Day 3 onwards).
- Prior to use, NidOil is temperature- and CO_2- equilibrated, but does not require washing or equilibration against culture medium.

Control mechanisms:

- Expiry dates are controlled, and the lot/batch number of each medium used recorded for every lab event on the lab forms and within the IDEAS database.
- Large bottles of NidOil are aliquoted into Falcon culture flasks for temperature pre-equilibration for ICSI; blastocyst culture dishes are pre-equilibrated overnight.
- NidOil requires storage at ambient temperature, and the temperature of the laboratory is monitored by the ReAssure system.

ICSI Products

Description:

- Hyaluronidase is used for stripping oocytes prior to ICSI. The Hyase10X™ product from Vitrolife (Göteborg, Sweden) is stored frozen at –20°C.
- Either PVP (ICSI™ from Vitrolife, stored at +2°C to +8°C) or SpermCatch (Nidacon, store unopened bottles at ambient temperature [+2°C to 30°C], once opened store at +2°C to 8°C) is used to slow the sperm for selection and catching for microinjection into oocytes.
- Microtools (holding and injection pipettes) are stored at ambient temperature.

Control mechanisms:

- Hyase and ICSI, and opened bottles of SpermCatch, are stored in the Embryology Lab fridge/freezer which is monitored by the ReAssure system.
- Unopened bottles of SpermCatch require storage at ambient temperature, and the temperature of the laboratory is monitored by the ReAssure system.
- Expiry dates are controlled, and the lot/batch number of each product recorded on the lab form and in the IDEAS database.

Culture dishes

Description: Various sizes and shapes of sterile plastic dishes for oocyte/zygote/embryo handling and culture. However, only dishes that fit properly in the bench-top incubators can be used.

Control mechanisms:

- Wherever possible use only MEA tested dishes.
- There have been very few verified reports over the past 30 years of specific gamete or embryo toxicity of Falcon or Nunc dishes, affording them a high degree of confidence worldwide. SparMed dishes are relatively new, but are of very high quality with extensive biocompatibility QC testing.
- Expiry dates are controlled, and the lot/batch number of each product recorded on the various lab forms and in the IDEAS database.
- Monitor the internet global forum EmbryoMail for problems, even perceived problems, with culture dishes.

Culture tubes

Description: Sterile round bottom polystyrene culture tubes from BD Falcon in 5 ml and 14 ml sizes (Falcon #2003 and #2001, respectively). The #2001 tubes are used to collect the follicular fluid aspirated at OPU.

Control mechanisms:

- There have been no verified reports over the past 30 years of specific gamete or embryo toxicity of Falcon tubes, affording them a high degree of confidence worldwide.

- Expiry dates are controlled, and the lot/batch number of each product recorded on the various lab forms and in the IDEAS database.

Centrifuge tubes

Description: Sterile conical bottom 15 ml polystyrene centrifuge tubes from BD Falcon are preferred; for polypropylene tubes, only ones that have been QC tested should be used.

Control mechanisms:

- There have been no verified reports over the past 30 years of specific spermotoxicity of Falcon polystyrene centrifuge tubes, affording them a high degree of confidence worldwide.
- SparMed polypropylene tubes are QC tested for possible toxicity.

Handling devices

Description:
- Glass Pasteur pipettes (e.g. Humagen, from Origio) are used during OPUs and sperm preparation.
- Cook Flexipets or Origio Strippers are used for stripping oocytes for ICSI, stripping presumptive zygotes after IVF, and handling stripped oocytes, zygotes and embryos.
- Disposable sterile plastic transfer pipettes are sometimes used during semen analysis and sperm preparation.

Control mechanisms:

- All products are specifically produced for IVF use and are MEA tested.
- While the soft plastic transfer pipettes are sterile they are not produced specifically for IVF, but are in common use.
- Expiry dates are controlled, and the lot/batch number of each product recorded on the various lab forms and within the IDEAS database.

OPU Needle Sets

Description: These sterile devices comprise a steel needle with attached plastic tubing and bung to fit the Falcon #2001 tubes.

Control mechanisms:

- Use only OPU needle sets that are manufactured specifically for this purpose, and QC tested for biocompatibility.
- Expiry dates should be controlled, and the lot/batch number of each product recorded on the lab ET form and in the IDEAS database.
- Monitor the internet global forum EmbryoMail for problems (even perceived problems).

Embryo transfer catheters

Description: Two-part (outer and inner) catheters for trans-cervical transfer of embryos into the uterus.

Control mechanisms:

- Use only catheters that are manufactured specifically for this purpose, and QC tested for biocompatibility.
- Expiry dates are controlled, and the lot/batch number of each product recorded on the lab form and in the IDEAS database.
- Monitor the internet global forum EmbryoMail for problems (even perceived problems).

Semen collection jars

Description: Sterile plastic jars without cardboard or rubber liners inside the lids (e.g. Starplex or SparMed Oosafe®).

Control mechanisms:

- Spermotoxicity has been tested under controlled conditions at various times over the past 30 years in numerous labs, with no evidence of adverse effects on sperm motility or vitality.
- We know of no verified reports over the past 30 years of specific spermotoxicity of StarPlex semen collection jars, affording them a high degree of confidence.
- SparMed jars are specifically QC tested for biocompatibility.
- Expiry dates are controlled, and the lot/batch number of this product recorded in the lab documentation and within the IDEAS database.

Culture flasks (for culture medium or oil aliquotting)

Description: Sterile polystyrene tissue culture flasks (50 ml and 250 ml sizes) from BD Falcon.

Control Mechanisms:

- There have been very few verified reports over the past 30 years of specific embryotoxicity of Falcon culture flasks, affording them a high degree of confidence worldwide.
- Expiry dates are controlled, and the lot/batch number of each product recorded in the lab documentation.

Serological pipettes

Description: Sterile polystyrene serological pipettes of various sizes from BD Falcon.

Control mechanisms:

- There have been no verified reports over the past 30 years of specific gamete or embryotoxicity of Falcon serological pipettes, affording them a high degree of confidence worldwide.

- Expiry dates are controlled, and the lot/batch number of each product recorded in the lab documentation.

Lab gases

Description: These gases are supplied by a specialist company and supplied to the equipment within the laboratories through reticulation systems (see "Equipment", below).

- *CO_2:* Supplied as medical grade 100% CO_2
- *Special mix:* Supplied as 6.0% CO_2/5.0% O_2/balance N_2 with certificates of assay provided with each medical grade cylinder. We use a "primary standard" grade of mixture, i.e. the two critical components will be within ±2.0% relative of the specific values (in this case, 5.88–6.12% CO_2 and 4.9–5.1% O_2).

Control mechanisms:

- All batch numbers are recorded and certificates of assay stored.
- The percentage CO_2 within the special mix gas can be verified using a hand-held i.r. CO_2 analyzer.

Sterile water

Description: Sterile water used to fill the humidity trays of the workstation and CO_2 incubator, as well as the humidification bottles of the BT37 incubators.

- Sterile water for irrigation (USP grade), from an established medical products manufacturer, with no antimicrobial agents added. The bottles might be of a "semi-rigid" plastic (polypropylene-based), but it should be pyrogen-, PVC- and DEHP-free.
- Bottles are pre-warmed to 37°C to avoid creating any cooling artefact when adding the water into temperature-controlled equipment.

Control mechanisms:

- Expiry dates are controlled, and the lot/batch number recorded in the lab documentation.

Equipment
Tube warmer

Description: Used to maintain the temperature of Falcon #2001 tubes as they are receiving the follicular fluid aspirates, e.g. Cook KFTH-1012.

Control mechanisms:

- Calibrated to maintain fluid contents of the Falcon #2001 tubes at 37 °C.
- Temperatures are logged manually since these units cannot be easily connected to the ReAssure system.
- Each unit is re-calibrated annually by the manufacturer or certified biomedical engineer.

Aspiration pump

Description: Used to create suction for aspirating follicular fluid and oocytes, e.g. Cook K-MAR.

- Should be used at ~100–110 mmHg suction pressure.

Control mechanisms:

- Aspiration suction pressure check is confirmed verbally before starting the procedure and noted on the surgical checklist (checkbox) by the procedural nurse.
- Each pump is re-calibrated annually by the manufacturer or certified biomedical engineer.

Workstation or "IVF chamber"

Description: The primary workstation for all handling of oocytes and embryos from OPU through to ET.

- Temperature controlled.
- CO_2 controlled (i.r. controller).
- Humidified (passive evaporation from a heated water tray).
- Incoming CO_2 passes through a built-in VOC filter as well as the one in the lab gas supply system.
- The internal air system needs to be re-circulating with built-in HEPA filtration.

Control mechanisms:

- The system has been calibrated to allow specimens to be maintained in the range of 35.0–37.5°C, and characterized so that useful working times are known for the different procedures.
- Display values for temperature and percentage CO_2 are logged at the start of each day by the duty embryologist.
- Temperature, humidity, and CO_2 are monitored using independent sensors connected to the ReAssure system.
- Separate verification of temperature and percentage CO_2 are also performed periodically using hand-held devices. The hand-held digital thermometer is calibrated in-house against a certified reference thermometer.

Andrology incubator

Description: A general-purpose air incubator used to maintain semen samples at 37°C during liquefaction. An orbital mixer is located inside the incubator to provide mixing of the ejaculates as they liquefy.

Control mechanisms:

- The incubator has been calibrated to maintain specimens at 37.0 ± 0.5°C.
- Display values for temperature are logged at the start of each day by the duty andrologist.

- Temperature is monitored using an independent sensor connected to the ReAssure system.
- Separate verification of temperature is also performed periodically using a hand-held digital thermometer that has been calibrated in-house against a certified reference thermometer.

Medium equilibration (CO_2-in-air) incubator

Description: A CO_2-in-air incubator located in the embryology lab used for the overnight pre-equilibration of culture dishes, e.g. Binder or Galaxy units.

- Temperature controlled.
- CO_2 controlled (i.r. controller).
- Humidified (passive evaporation from a water tray).
- Incoming CO_2 is VOC filtered in the lab gas supply system.

Control mechanisms:

- The incubator has been calibrated to maintain dishes at $37.0 \pm 0.5°C$.
- Display values for temperature and percentage CO_2 are logged at the start of each day by the duty embryologist.
- Temperature, humidity, and CO_2 are monitored using independent sensors connected to the ReAssure system.
- Separate verification of temperature and percentage CO_2 are also performed periodically using hand-held devices. The hand-held digital thermometer is calibrated in-house against a certified reference thermometer.

Embryo culture incubators

Description: Compact bench-top incubators (Planer BT37) for fertilization and embryo culture that use pre-mixed gas.

- Temperature calibrated with the base of each dish sitting in direct contact with the substantial thermal mass to ensure the most rapid re-equilibration of incubation temperature with minimal fluctuations.
- Gas flow controlled, including a purge mode after each opening to flush air out of the incubation compartments and ensure the most rapid restitution of the proper atmosphere (6.0% CO_2/5.0% O_2/balance N_2).

Control mechanisms:

- The incubator is calibrated to maintain specimens at $37°C$.
- Display values for temperature are logged at the start of each day by the duty embryologist.
- Temperature is monitored using an independent sensor connected to the ReAssure system.
- The internal data logging of each incubator is also logged by the ReAssure system.
- Separate verification of temperature is also performed periodically using a hand-held digital thermometer that has been calibrated in-house against a certified reference thermometer.

ICSI rig

Description: For example, an Olympus IX71 inverted microscope with relief contrast optics and a Tokai Hit ThermoPlate glass heated stage insert. Narishige micromanipulators and microinjectors are attached, as well as a Hamilton Thorne LYKOS laser system and Research Instruments Viewer digital imaging software.

Control mechanisms:

- The ThermoPlate heated stage has been calibrated to maintain the contents of culture dishes at 37.0°C.
- Display values for temperature are logged at the start of each day, and for each ICSI procedure, by the duty embryologist.
- Temperature is monitored using an independent sensor connected to the ReAssure system.
- Separate verification of temperature is also performed periodically using a hand-held digital thermometer that has been calibrated in-house against a certified reference thermometer.

Refrigerator–freezer

Description: A domestic-grade combined refrigerator-freezer used for storing various materials including stock and ready-use supplies of culture media and related products.

Control mechanisms:

- Temperatures are set to maintain ranges of below −20°C in the freezer compartments and +4°C to +8°C in the refrigerator compartments.
- Display values for local digital thermometer readings on internal temperatures are logged at the start of each day by the duty andrologist or embryologist. These digital thermometers have been calibrated in-house against a certified reference thermometer.
- Independent temperature sensors are installed in both the refrigerator and freezer compartments that are connected to the ReAssure system. Door-opening sensors are also fitted and connected to the ReAssure system.
- Separate independent verification of temperature is also performed periodically using a hand-held digital thermometer that has been calibrated in-house against a certified reference thermometer.

Vertical laminar flow cabinets (VLAFs)

Description: Workstations used for handling sperm during washing, gametes and embryos during freezing and thawing, and also when preparing culture dishes, that protect the specimens from contamination by the operator. Air inside the cabinets is HEPA filtered to achieve ISO Class 4 or better (GMP Grade A).

Note: Class II biohazard cabinets should be used when handling semen samples.

Control mechanisms:

- All VLAF cabinets are certified by a specialized company as meeting the required standard; re-certification is repeated on an annual basis.

- In-house measurement of particulates inside the cabinets using a hand-held particle counter typically shows zero values.

Gas reticulation system

Description: For each gas used to supply incubation systems (e.g. CO_2, special mix, nitrogen for tri-gas incubators, compressed air for anti-vibration tables):
- Two banks of $2 \times K$ size cylinders connected to an autochange manifold.
- An autochange manifold to switch over to the other pair of cylinders when the supply pressure drops below a pre-set limit.
- A gas control panel that shows an alert following cylinder bank switching so that the lab staff can replace the empty cylinders, and an alarm state should the changeover fail.
- After the autochange manifold the gas flows through a VOC extraction filter (two are connected in parallel so that they can be swapped without needing to interrupt the gas supply to the lab) and is then distributed through stainless steel piping to the various connection points throughout the lab suite where equipment is connected via Swagelok QuickConnect devices.

Control mechanisms:

- Gas cylinder pressures are noted at the start and end of each day by lab staff and logged on the daily checklist.
- All cylinders of special mix gas are "primary standard" quality and come with a certificate of assay to confirm the correct composition.
- The gas control panel will alert lab staff to any issues with the autochange units and supply pressures. Under-pressure alerts are connected to the ReAssure system to trigger alarm conditions.

Lab processes
Pre-OPU [Day −1]

Description:
- Dishes for the OPU, as well as IVF or ICSI procedures, that contain fertilization medium (bicarbonate-buffered) are prepared the afternoon before and equilibrated for temperature and CO_2 overnight in a CO_2 incubator.
- Adequate supplies of dishes and Pasteur pipettes within the IVF workstation are verified.
- Tubes of gamete buffer (HEPES-buffered) are tight-capped and placed in an incubator to equilibrate for temperature.

Control mechanisms:

- Display temperatures, and percentage CO_2 values where controlled by the incubator, are recorded on the embryology daily checklist.
- The ReAssure system monitors and logs critical incubator conditions every 5 minutes.

OPU [Day 0]

Description:
This procedure integrates both clinical and laboratory aspects.
- The workstation is at the required temperature and its humidity tray filled with water.
- The patient's vagina is cleaned using sterile saline; gametotoxic solutions (such as chlorhexidine or betadine) are not used.
- Follicular fluid is aspirated at ~100–110 mmHg negative pressure into sterile round bottom culture tubes. The tubing connecting the needle to the tubes is an integral part of the needle set supplied by Cook. The tubing connecting the downstream side of the tube to the suction pump is re-usable, but does not come into contact with the follicular fluid or oocytes.
- Collection tubes are pre-warmed and held in the tube warmer while they are being filled. Tubes are then transferred essentially immediately to the workstation through the tube rack port.
- Tube contents (follicular aspirates) are tipped into 60 mm dishes for "egg search"; identified COCs are washed through a "rinse" dish and transferred to the "OPU" dish. After grading, at the end of the OPU all COCs are transferred into the "insemination" dish and transferred to a bench-top incubator until insemination (IVF or ICSI).

Control mechanisms:

All efforts must be made to maintain oocytes within the temperature range of 35.0–37.5°C, and protected from pH shifts by using a CO_2-enriched atmosphere.
- Aspiration suction pressure check is part of the mandatory surgical checklist; it is confirmed verbally (as with patient ID) before starting the procedure and noted on the surgical checklist by the procedural nurse.
- The tube warmer's temperature is monitored and logged as part of the lab's daily checklist (since it is not practicable to connect it to the ReAssure system).
- Workstation operation (temperature, RH and percentage CO_2) is monitored and logged.
- To minimize any possible effect of temperature shifts within the workstation (e.g. evaporative cooling artefact) all egg-search and washing procedures are performed quickly, within pre-defined time limits; achieving this speed is an integral element of defining embryologist competence.
- Assessments employ a standardized grading scheme that facilitates rapid recording of the observations, minimizing the total time required.
- Dishes containing fertilization medium (bicarbonate-buffered) are prepared the afternoon before and equilibrated overnight for temperature and CO_2.
- COCs are assessed using a standardized grading scheme that facilitates rapid recording of the observations, minimizing the total time required.

Sperm preparation [Day 0]

Description:
- A semen sample is collected by the male partner ideally after the OPU and incubated at 37°C with orbital mixing inside an air incubator in the andrology lab.

- As soon as possible after the sample has liquefied (typically ~20 min) analysis and preparation/washing are commenced. Washing uses a pair of PureSperm discontinuous density gradients (prepared using Gamete Buffer to avoid pH shifts) with centrifugation at 300 g × 20 min. Pellet recovery from the bottom of the gradient tubes is performed very carefully to minimize possible contamination with seminal plasma or other semen components.
- Pellets are combined and washed using Gamete Buffer with centrifugation at 500 g × 10 min.
- The washed sperm suspension is prepared in Gamete Buffer except for IVF cases where insemination will be performed within 2 hours when they are re-suspended directly into fertilization medium.
- ICSI samples in Gamete Buffer are held at ambient temperature in the dark to minimize possible oxidative damage.
- IVF samples prepared more than two hours before insemination are also held in gamete buffer at ambient temperature in the dark to prevent premature capacitation and possible burn-out, as well as minimizing possible oxidative damage. About two hours before insemination time they are washed into fertilization medium and then incubated at 37°C in a CO_2-enriched atmosphere (CO_2-in-air incubator) to promote capacitation.

Control mechanisms:

- The centrifuges are programmed to prevent incorrect centrifugation speed/time combinations.
- Correct, careful techniques for running and harvesting gradients and for washing sperm are defined in the relevant SOPs and observance of all details is inherent to defining competence of anyone performing the procedure.
- Temperature and percentage CO_2 of the CO_2-in-air incubator are logged and monitored as described above; proper operation of the bench-top incubators is logged and monitored.

IVF insemination [Day 0]

Description:
- The "insem" dish is taken from the bench-top incubator to the workstation; the sperm prep tube is taken from the CO_2-in-air incubator to the workstation.
- The sperm prep tube is mixed and the required volume of sperm suspension added to each well of the "insem" dish.
- The "insem" dish is taken from the workstation and returned to the bench-top incubator.

Control mechanisms:

Protect oocytes from adverse temperature and pH_e.
- Minimize possible cooling of the oocytes to 35°C or below, or pH shift of the fertilization medium (caused by exposure to air for 2 min).
- Distance between the bench-top incubators and the workstation has been minimized by lab layout; time required is only a few seconds.

- Temperature and CO_2 are controlled within the workstation while the "insem" dish is opened for sperm addition.
- Proper operation of the bench-top incubators and workstation are logged and monitored.

ICSI [Day 0]

Description:

- The "insem" dish is taken from the bench-top incubator to the workstation.
- Oocytes are stripped of their cumulus and corona cells using hyaluronidase inside the workstation.
- The "ICSI" dish prepared with droplets containing the stripped oocytes and prepared sperm inside the workstation.
- The ICSI dish is transferred to the ICSI rig (e.g. inverted microscope with Tokai Hit ThermoPlate heated insert and Narishige micromanipulators and microinjectors).
- ICSI is performed.
- ICSI dish is taken back to the workstation and injected oocytes transferred into the "post-ICSI" dish, which is then replaced in a bench-top incubator for overnight fertilization culture.

Control mechanisms:

Protect oocytes from adverse temperature and pH_e.

- Minimize possible cooling of the oocytes to 35°C or below, or pH shift of the fertilization medium (caused by exposure to air for 2 min).
- Distance between the bench-top incubators and the workstation has been minimized by lab layout; time required is only a few seconds.
- For the "insem" and "post-ICSI" dishes, temperature and CO_2 are controlled within the workstation, where the dishes are opened for removal or replacement of oocytes before/after injection.
- Distance between the workstation and ICSI rig is minimized by lab layout; the time required is only a few seconds.
- The temperature of the ICSI dish on the ICSI rig is maintained by the stage warmer since it has been previously established that a dummy ICSI dish on the microscope heated stage experiences minor temperature loss (0.3°C) over a 5 min period (operation of the stage warmer is logged and monitored). The medium pH in the ICSI drops is maintained by the HEPES buffer of the Gamete Buffer medium used.
- Proper operation of the bench-top incubators and workstation are logged and monitored.

Fertilization culture [Days 0–1]

Description:

Inseminated oocytes (using either IVF or ICSI) are cultured in fertilization medium overnight in a bench-top incubator.

Control mechanisms:

Protect oocytes from adverse temperature and pH_e.

- Proper operation of the bench-top incubators is logged and monitored by the ReAssure system.
- Proper pCO_2 (and low O_2) is achieved continuously via a supply of pre-mixed gas.

Preparation for cleavage culture [Day 0]

Description:
The cleavage dish is prepared on the afternoon of Day 0 and equilibrated for temperature and CO_2 overnight in a CO_2 incubator (bench-top or CO_2-in-air incubator).

Control mechanisms:

- Display temperatures (and percentage CO_2 value if controlled by the incubator) are recorded on the embryology daily checklist.
- The ReAssure system monitors and logs critical incubator conditions continuously.

Fertilization check [Day 1]

Description:
Examine oocytes at 17 ± 1 h post-insemination/ICSI for evidence of fertilization.

- The "insem" or "post-ICSI" dish is transferred from the bench-top incubator to the workstation; the "cleavage" dish is transferred from the equilibration incubator into the workstation.
- For IVF cases, any remaining cumulus and corona cells are removed from the oocyte using Strippers or Flexipets; this is not necessary for ICSI cases since oocytes were stripped prior to injection.
- Presumptive zygotes are examined under the stereozoom microscope for signs of fertilization.
- Detailed observations typically require the use of the inverted (ICSI) microscope. If this cannot be performed within a maximum period of two minutes exposure to room air atmosphere then transfer the oocytes/zygotes into an observation dish containing temperature-equilibrated Gamete Buffer to protect them during the time they will be exposed to room air.
- Upon completing the assessment, the culture dish is transferred from the inverted microscope back into the workstation (if necessary) and the zygotes moved into the cleavage dish and returned to a bench-top incubator.

Control mechanisms:

Protect the presumptive zygotes from adverse temperature and pH_e.

- Minimize possible cooling of the oocytes to 35°C or below, or pH shift of the fertilization medium (caused by exposure to air for 2 min).
- The distance between the bench-top incubators and the workstation is minimized by lab layout; the time required is only a few seconds.

- Temperature and CO_2 for the insem and cleavage dishes are controlled within the workstation while (presumptive) zygotes are being assessed and transferred into ongoing culture.
- Proper operation of the workstation is logged and monitored.
- The distance between the workstation and the inverted microscope is minimized by lab layout; the time required is only a few seconds.
- During any assessments performed on the inverted microscope, temperature is maintained by a stage warmer since it has been previously established that a dummy ICSI dish on the microscope heated stage only experiences minor temperature loss (0.3°C) over a 5 min period (operation of the stage warmer is logged and monitored). The medium pH of the drops is maintained either by taking less than 2 min, or by the HEPES buffer of the Gamete Buffer in an observation dish.
- Zygote assessments employ a standardized grading scheme that facilitates rapid recording of the observations, minimizing the total time required.

Embryo culture [Days 1–5 or 6]

Description:
Embryos are cultured in cleavage medium from Day 1 through early Day 3, and blastocyst medium from the morning of Day 3 onwards, in a bench-top incubator.

Control mechanisms:

Protect embryos from adverse temperature and pH_e.

- Proper operation of the bench-top incubators is logged and monitored by the ReAssure system.
- Proper pCO_2 (and low O_2) is achieved continuously via a supply of pre-mixed gas.

Embryo assessments [Days 2–5]

Description:
Examination of embryos at the following time points (defined in hours post-insemination or "*p-i*", as per the Istanbul Consensus 2011) for assessment of development rate and grading:

1. Cleavage stage embryos: Day 2 @ 44 ± 1 h *p-i*; Day 3 @ 68 ± 1 h *p-i*
2. Morula stage embryos: Day 4 @ 92 ± 2 h *p-i*
3. Blastocyst stage embryos: Day 5 @ 116 ± 2 h *p-i*; Day 6 @ 140 ± 2 h *p-i*
- The "cleavage" or "blast" embryo culture dish is transferred from the bench-top incubator to the workstation.
- Embryos are examined under the stereozoom microscope.
- Detailed observations typically require the use of the inverted (ICSI) microscope. If this cannot be performed within a maximum period of 2 min exposure to room air atmosphere then transfer the embryos into an observation dish containing temperature-equilibrated Gamete Buffer to protect them during the time they will be under room air.

- Upon completing the assessment, the embryo culture dish is transferred from the inverted microscope back into the workstation (if necessary) and the embryos moved back into the culture dish and returned to a bench-top incubator.

Control mechanisms:

Protect the embryos from adverse temperature and pH_e.

- Protect against possible cooling of the embryos to 35°C or below, or pH shift of the cleavage medium or blastocyst medium, as appropriate (caused by exposure to air for 2 min).
- The distance between the bench-top incubators and the workstation is minimized by lab layout; the transit time required is only a few seconds.
- The temperature and CO_2 for the cleavage and blast dishes are controlled within the workstation while embryos are being assessed.
- Proper operation of the workstation is logged and monitored.
- The distance between the workstation and inverted microscope is minimized by lab layout; the time required is only a few seconds.
- During any assessments performed on the inverted microscope, the temperature is maintained by a stage warmer since it has been previously established that a dummy ICSI dish on the microscope heated stage only experiences minor temperature loss (0.3°C) over a 5 min period (operation of the stage warmer is logged and monitored). The medium pH of the drops is maintained either by taking less than 2 min, or by the HEPES buffer of the Gamete Buffer in an observation dish.
- Embryo assessments employ a standardized grading scheme that facilitates rapid recording of the observations, minimizing the total time required.

Preparation for extended culture [Day 2]

Description:
  A "blast" dish is prepared on the afternoon of Day 2 and equilibrated for temperature and CO_2 overnight in a CO_2 incubator (bench-top or CO_2-in-air incubator). If culture is to be prolonged to Day 6 then a second blast dish must be prepared on the afternoon of Day 4 because culture medium needs to be replaced after each 48 hours of culture.

Control mechanisms:

- Display temperatures (and percentage CO_2 value if controlled by the incubator) are recorded on the embryology daily checklist.
- The ReAssure system monitors and logs critical incubator conditions continuously.

Extended culture [Days 3–5]

Description:
  Normally performed in combination with the Day 3 embryo assessment.
- The "cleavage" dish is transferred from the bench-top incubator to the workstation; the "blast" dish is transferred from the equilibration incubator into the workstation.

- Embryos are examined under the stereozoom microscope.
- Detailed observations typically require the use of the inverted (ICSI) microscope. If this cannot be performed within a maximum period of 2 min then transfer the embryos into an observation dish containing temperature-equilibrated Gamete Buffer to protect them during the time they will be under the room air atmosphere.
- Upon completing the assessment, embryos are transferred into the blast dish and returned to a bench-top incubator.

Control mechanisms:

Protect the embryos from adverse temperature and pH_e.

- Protect against possible cooling of the embryos to 35°C or below, or pH shift of the cleavage medium or blastocyst medium, as appropriate (caused by exposure to air for 2 min).
- The distance between the bench-top incubators and the workstation is minimized by lab layout; the time required is only a few seconds.
- The temperature and CO_2 for the cleavage and blast dishes are controlled within the workstation while embryos are being assessed.
- Proper operation of the workstation is logged and monitored.
- The distance between the workstation and inverted microscope is minimized by lab layout; the time required is only a few seconds.
- During any assessments performed on the inverted microscope, the temperature is maintained by a stage warmer since it has been previously established that a dummy ICSI dish on the microscope heated stage only experiences minor temperature loss (0.3°C) over a 5 min period (operation of the stage warmer is logged and monitored). The medium pH of the drops is maintained either by taking less than 2 min, or by the HEPES buffer of the Gamete Buffer in an observation dish.
- Embryo assessments employ a standardized grading scheme that facilitates rapid recording of the observations, minimizing the total time required.

Preparation for embryo transfer [usually Day 2 or 4]

Description:

An ET dish is prepared on the afternoon of the day before the ET procedure and equilibrated for temperature and CO_2 in a CO_2 incubator overnight (bench-top or CO_2-in-air incubator). Cleavage medium is used for cleavage stage embryo transfers (i.e. Day 3), blastocyst medium for blastocyst stage transfers (i.e. Day 5 or 6).

Control mechanisms:

- Display temperatures (and percentage CO_2 value if controlled by the incubator) are recorded on the embryology daily checklist.
- The ReAssure system monitors and logs critical incubator conditions continuously.

Embryo transfer [usually Day 3 or 5]

Description:

This procedure includes both clinical and laboratory aspects; both have been included here for completeness.

- The workstation is at the required temperature and percentage CO_2, and its humidity tray filled with water.
- The patient's vagina is cleaned using sterile saline; embryotoxic solutions (e.g. chlorhexidine, betadine) are *not* used, and cervical mucus is removed carefully.
- The "cleavage" or "blast" embryo culture dish is transferred from the bench-top incubator to the workstation; the "ET" dish is transferred from the equilibration incubator into the workstation.
- Embryos are examined under the stereozoom microscope.
- The embryo(s) to be transferred is/are moved into the ET dish and the embryo culture dish replaced in the bench-top incubator until later.
- The embryo(s) to be transferred is/are shown to the procedure room via the video link.
- At the appropriate juncture the embryo(s) is/are loaded into the catheter, which is then taken into the procedure room and handed to the clinician.
- After the clinician has performed the ET, the catheter is taken back into the workstation in the lab and checked for returned embryos.

Control Mechanisms:

Protect the embryos from adverse temperature and pH_e.

- Protect against possible cooling of the embryos to 35°C or below, or pH shift of the cleavage medium or blastocyst medium, as appropriate (caused by exposure to air for 2 min).
- The distance between the bench-top incubators and the workstation is minimized by lab layout; the time required is only a few seconds.
- The temperature and CO_2 for the cleavage, blast, and ET dishes are controlled within the workstation while embryos are being handled and assessed.
- Proper operation of the workstation is logged and monitored.
- The distance between the workstation and the procedure room table is minimized by lab layout; the time required is only a few seconds.

Is the "well-run lab" enough?: quality and risk management in the IVF clinic

We hope that the preceding chapters will have provided sufficient background and introduction to the tools and techniques used in quality management and risk management to allow any IVF lab director to embark upon the road towards becoming the best IVF lab in the world. This is not a facetious remark: everyone has access to the same protocols, equipment, techniques, training, plasticware, culture media, etc., as anyone else – so why shouldn't any lab, anywhere, have the same opportunity to be as good as any other?

But why would we want to expend what is, unarguably, a huge amount of effort, on changing the nice comfortable lab that we've been running for *n* years into one that will require us to spend a not inconsiderable amount of time monitoring and dealing with all the QC/QA issues, document control, etc.? To our minds, the explanation can be summed up as:

1. Being professional: the need to always do one's best and adhere to the principle of *primum non nocere*; and
2. The advantages: better results, less risks, higher morale, and confidence.

For those working in the private sector then the commercial advantage of improved success rates must also be factored into the equation.

But even if we've convinced you of the importance of effective quality and risk management in the IVF lab, what about the IVF clinic as a whole? Is it worth investing the same sort of time and effort into adopting a total quality management approach everywhere? In this chapter, we will work through a cost–benefit analysis of taking a quality approach, and make some suggestions about where to start.

Does quality "cost" or "pay"?

The "ideal" ART program is one that has lots of patient referrals, a good take-home baby rate, with a low incidence of complications, and satisfied staff who feel like valued members of a team. It is financially stable, and has good communication, both internally between staff and externally with patients and referrers. It will collect and use data for process management, and planning, and embrace the concept of continuous quality improvement. This might sound so idealistic as to be unachievable, but we have had the pleasure of observing and managing clinics that had all of these characteristics, as a result of their quality management system.

So what are the characteristics we have observed in the absence of a quality management system? In those clinics that run "organically," using the same approach they have used since their start-up phase, there is often uncontrolled risk in all facets of operation, which can result in extreme adverse incidents. Furthermore, there are generally unpredictable outcomes, due to a lack of process control, with wide, random variations in process that can lead to "system crashes." As a result, there is a lot of time spent in troubleshooting – correcting apparently random errors and putting out "fires" that seem to arise spontaneously (i.e. with no specific identifiable root cause). This can lead to a pervasive atmosphere of "drama" across the clinic, where even relatively minor problems are seen to be disproportionately large and critical. Over time, staff members become disengaged from the mission of the clinic, as they perceive the workplace to be toxic, and they become disinterested in new approaches or opportunities for improvement. This leads to high rates of staff turnover, leading to a loss of corporate memory and a shortage of content experts. This is a depressing picture, and of course not all clinics without a formal quality management system have all of these attributes – but sadly, most have at least some. Fortunately, by recognizing that there is the opportunity for change, many of these problems can be addressed.

Implementing a quality management system does have some associated costs, and these are not trivial – although the majority of the financial investment required is a "one-off." These costs are related to:

- A database/enhanced EMR system
- Real-time logging system(s)
- A system for "witnessing" lab procedures
- Independent measuring devices for laboratory QC (such as certified calibration thermometers)
- Enrolment in EQC/EQA schemes (lab and clinical).

However, it is possible to mitigate some of these costs. For example, a competent database system is used to manage patient information, thereby reducing or removing the staff costs associated with searching for paper-based charts, and reducing risk by ensuring that copies of signed consents are available to the relevant clinic personnel when and where they need to see them. Because all data are entered into the database when they are generated, this reduces multiple handling of the same data (saving time and typos). Having all the data in one place means that extra staff time is not required to generate reports on outcome statistics (such as those required by national registries and/or regulatory bodies) and KPIs, as the database should be able to provide these reports automatically. Together, these represent perfect examples of waste that can be eliminated by taking a quality management approach (as discussed in Chapter 3).

Similarly, the hardware cost of a real-time logging system (as discussed in Chapters 11 and 13) can be recovered within two years regardless of clinic size, based on time recovered by not having to do the independent measurements of temperature, CO_2, etc. for equipment QC (as must be done in any well-run lab). A bonus is that records can be created as often as once every five minutes, rather than once or twice a day, as for the manual system.

Other ongoing costs are related to staff time in collecting data for monitoring, the need for strong leadership and commitment to the philosophy of quality management, and the need to educate and mentor staff through the associated change process. In larger clinics, there might also be the expense of hiring a full-time quality manager.

Against these costs, there are a number of benefits associated with having a quality management system in place. For example, effective process management reduces both outcome variability and the need for troubleshooting, as many of the risks that lead to system failures have been mitigated or controlled. This in turn leads to improved efficiency in all areas of the clinic, since there is a reduced requirement for "re-work" to correct mistakes, which has the additional benefit of encouraging staff to remain engaged and interested. Together, these result in improved success rates, which is the reason that patients come to the clinic in the first place.

A bonus of having a fully functional quality management system is that the preparation for accreditation is not an "extra" one to two year project for which extra time must be found. Rather, it might be as simple as completing a self-assessment questionnaire, since all of the aspects that are surveyed are already under control. Also, when setting up a quality management system, it is not necessary to do it from scratch. Seek advice from other clinics or other experts, but then tailor it to fit your clinic to truly reflect the way you do things – in much the same way as you do when adapting SOPs.

A quality approach to resource management

In any business, it is imperative to balance resource use with income, and to ensure that resources are not squandered. It is possible to utilize a quality approach to resource management, with the same positive outcomes that may be seen in the laboratory. In addition to money, resources that must be managed are:

- Time
- Human resources
- Information
- Good-will and reputation.

Time and money

In a quality program the processes are all mapped, so:

- The number and type of referrals is known and can be projected;
- The range of procedures, and the number of each is known; and
- The time and costs for each procedure should also be known.

Taken together, this information can be used to develop a business model with a standard operating budget, projection of the number of people needed for workload, creation of standing orders with suppliers (which results in significant cost savings across the year and is the best guarantee of supply), and the ability to forecast the impact of new opportunities or threats. This supports the financial stability, and ongoing stability of the clinic, enhancing good-will and reputation.

Human resources

As discussed in Chapter 12, managing human resources well is critical to a successful IVF laboratory, and IVF clinic. It is critical to avoid the "toxic workplace" trap of taking staff and their loyalty and commitment/professional dedication for granted – or perhaps worse, of assuming that people will put up with anything in exchange for a regular pay check. Managing your human resources requires building trust. Because the quality improvement cycle is based on making meaningful improvements to the system, a quality environment is one in which change is always occurring. Since people most want to know that their contribution to their workplace is valuable and valued, the key to managing change, and promoting the concept of quality, is recognizing the need for open communication, with honesty and respect on both sides.

Information

The need for a smooth flow of information between different areas of the clinic, and between the clinic and its patients and referrers, cannot be overestimated. Quite simply, that flow of relevant information is the lifeblood of the clinic, reducing the risk that tasks might be overlooked or notifications forgotten. This does mean that everyone who has a piece of information must take responsibility for entering it into the database and/or patient's chart, as the integrity of the system is reliant upon this.

Good-will and reputation

A quality organization knows who its customers are, and recognizes their importance to its success. When all of the other resources are managed (time, money, and people), the organization is able to run smoothly. This enhances positive outcomes for patients and therefore the clinic's reputation with its peers, as well as with its patients and referrers.

What does it take?

To develop a quality clinic that achieves the highest success rates and minimizes its risks requires a broad spectrum of resources, a shortfall in any one of which can cause the whole endeavor to fail.

1. For any organization to be able to change, there is an absolute need for "slack" (DeMarco, 2001). Insufficient slack will compromise the availability of vital human resources and the stress on the morale of critical personnel will destroy their commitment to the process of change.

2. Everyone in the organization must be committed and involved. Involvement and support from the highest to the lowest members of the organization are vital, as is strong leadership.

3. Adequate resources: time and money. This might require additional personnel, some permanent, but many can be employed on a temporary basis or out-sourced as consultants.

4. The ability to manage change must exist within the organization (Heller and Hindle, 2003). All key players must understand human nature – our innate fear of change and the inertia that this creates.

5. Attitudes must be corrected where necessary: any culture of blame must be eliminated; mistakes must be seen as opportunities for improvement, not events that require scapegoats and punishment. There must be recognition that improvements are not a criticism of how things were done previously. People should be confident in speaking their minds, and feel confident in their own abilities. Basically, any element of a "toxic workplace" must be eradicated (Coombs, 2001).

6. A vision of how things should be run to create a positive environment for one's staff as well as focusing on what your "customers" want.

In Chapter 3 we discussed the change in perspective from being a "product-out" company to a "market-in" company that is focused on its customers. So while the typical

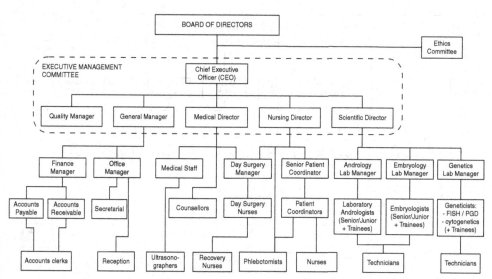

Figure 14.1 An organization chart for an IVF clinic reflecting the traditional ("product-out") view of its hierarchy, defining lines of authority and responsibility.

organizational chart for an IVF center shown in Figure 14.1 might serve the organization very well in terms of establishing its hierarchy and the lines of authority and responsibility, the alternative view of the same organization shown in Figure 14.2 eloquently illustrates the change in focus when a "market-in" organization provides its services.

How do we get there?

Achieving excellence in the IVF lab also requires the scientists who work there to think and act as scientists. As has been seen numerous times throughout this book, scientific method is at the foundation of many of the concepts and approaches used in quality management and risk management, and so we as scientists should see these areas as logical extensions of our scientific work and their achievement as being based on common sense. A valuable resource that we have found not only highly enjoyable to read, but a wonderful expression of what it takes to be a scientist is the book by Jack Cohen and Graham Medley entitled *Stop Working and Start Thinking: A Guide to Becoming a Scientist* (Cohen and Medley, 2005) – everyone working in a lab anywhere should read their book.

There are no short-cuts to achieving excellence, but a bird's-eye perspective of the "road map" is shown in Figure 14.3, the general concepts of which should be pretty familiar by now.

1. *Establish the goals* and get "buy-in" from everyone in the organization. This buy-in must be reinforced along the way, any setbacks or unresolved problems will create doubt in some of your people's minds, and once someone has lost faith in the process it's very much harder to get them back on board.

2. *Educate everyone* in the tools and techniques that will be used:
   a. Systems analysis and process mapping (including the flow charting tools that will be used);
   b. Benchmarking;

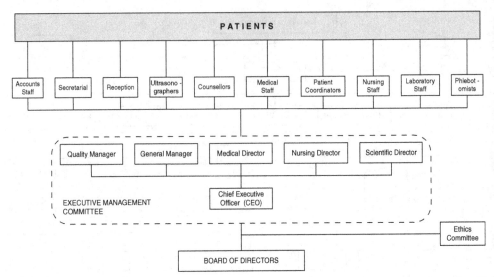

Figure 14.2 An alternate view of the organization chart for an IVF clinic that is focused on becoming a "market-in" company, more responsive to the needs of its patients.

    c. Audits;

    d. How to perform FMEAs and RCAs; and

    e. Scientific method and troubleshooting.

3. *Design the process* of what you will be doing:

    a. Appoint a quality manager;

    b. Ensure that management recognizes that the time spent by everyone working in their teams is counted as work time (including overtime, if required), and not personal time;

    c. Identify the areas for change and prioritize them (you can't change everything at once);

    d. Define the specific goals; and then

    e. Set a realistic timetable.

4. *Build the teams* who will tackle each of the areas:

    a. Identify the team leaders (*not* necessarily managers);

    b. Recruit the team members; and

    c. Have each team establish their scope of activities.

5. *Define* the areas for change:

    a. Each team reviews their area and identifies the initial targets for improvement;

    b. Each team then prioritizes their areas for change in terms of "bang for the buck" and risk minimization; and then

    c. Each team sets their goals, constructs the tasks that will lead to those goals, and identifies how each change will be monitored for effective implementation and efficacy (i.e. select Indicators) – in other words, they build their action plan.

6. *Implement* the changes contained in the action plan(s).

7. *Monitor* the changes using the defined indicators.

8. *Review* the outcomes – and then *revise* or *repeat* as necessary until the goal is achieved.

9. *Continue the cycle* because no system ever achieves perfection. This is the foundation of TQM and the underlying principle of all accreditation schemes.

In all of this, it is critical that an environment be created in which all members of staff feel able to buy into the process. This requires their direct involvement, so, for example, the role of the IVF lab director is not to run the whole TQM program for the lab. While the lab director might well lead one or more of the lab teams, (s)he will also be involved in teams working in other areas of the center, so would not have time to run all the teams. Allowing staff members to take a more active role also provides opportunities for career and personal development.

In any well-run IVF center the lab director must be a central, key figure in the organization. The lab cannot be "marginalized" and seen as just a "back room" where "the techs do their thing" – IVF does not exist without the lab and its people. Indeed, at the Alpha Foundation Workshop held during the 1999 World IVF Congress in Sydney, Bob Edwards opened the day with an uplifting perspective on the role of the scientist in ART, in which he made the point that IVF clinics should be run by scientists, while still emphasizing the importance of the team approach and mutual respect. At the conclusion of the talk he stated that scientists should be more able to understand business and finance (the better to run IVF programs) and suggested that Alpha or national clinical embryologist groups should consider providing business training as part of their educational remit. Throughout this presentation he emphasized that it is the scientist, not the clinician, who does science. Yet again, we marvel at the prescience of Bob Edwards, whose understanding of the field of scientific endeavor that he created is being vindicated by the increasing importance of the central role played by the IVF lab in accreditation and regulatory schemes.

Strategic planning

Getting the process started requires a significant amount of planning – but how many of us have sat through "strategic planning workshops," often taking up days of time (and so often at weekends...) that have generated impressive documents that will light the clinic's way forward through the next five years?

And how many of us have seen those ambitious plans fizzle and lead nowhere?

In this section we will briefly consider not how to create a strategic plan – because this is really no different to so many other quality exercises – but take the converse (perverse?) view: why do such plans fail? The software company SmartDraw, whose tagline is "Communicate Visually," have numerous white papers on their website, as well as running a corporate blog. A recent insightful article considered "10 Ways to Kill Your Strategic Plan" (Wilson, 2014):

1. *Lack of total team commitment*: basically failure to get buy-in from the entire staff will result in a lack of shared vision and a lack of commitment – without which even the best strategic plan is foredoomed. But achieving this must be through voluntary involvement, forced participation in change (worse still, required participation under threat) will not only be superficial, it will probably be counter-productive and perhaps even deadly to the entire plan. Effective teamwork requires leaders not managers (see Chapter 12).

2. *Not getting the right people involved*: without the involvement of those who are crucial to expounding the clinic's vision, and those who are responsible for its realization –

basically pretty well everyone in an IVF clinic – how can progress be made? Failing to involve a key stakeholder in the planning process can easily make that person feel disconnected (undermining team buy-in and commitment) and then either they, or those to whom they should have delegated the action steps, might well leave a critical element unaddressed.

3. *Failing to focus on the big picture*: strategic planning is, by its nature, intended to focus on high-level ideas. Not just wordsmithing the clinic's vision, mission, and goals statements, or dreaming up a new tagline, but real, actionable major issues that are critical to the clinic's future success.

4. *Not making an honest assessment of the present situation*: don't look at the clinic through your own eyes, or how you think others see you (so often this is no more than simply re-stating how you want yourself to be seen) – get an honest perspective from outside, collate and analyze your non-conformity reports (assuming you've allowed an honest, unfettered system of reporting to flourish), read the comments patients post in their support groups' chat rooms, use one or more focus groups of patients (and not just ones who got pregnant), and even commission a critical report from an independent consultant. Without an honest assessment of where you are, any strategic plan will be flawed, if not fundamentally compromised.

5. *Failure to consider the realities around you*: again, it's a matter of being honest. A clinic needs to not only be open to criticism of its services, but also perceptive of what's happening within "the market" and society at large. Patient expectations are market forces, but so are improved services and outcomes by your competitors, as well as societal factors such as the local economy and regulatory aspects of ART. Clinic management must be acutely aware of these factors on an ongoing basis, aware of how they might impact the clinic's operations, its customers (both patients and referrers), and the clinic's future.

6. *Unwillingness to change*: resistance to change is an inherent human trait, and everyone committed to quality must strive against it – not just in others, but within themselves. Any clinic, even one in the public sector, must continuously assess what's happening in the field of ART, and be ready and able to adapt; fighting against the need for change, or worse still, ignoring it entirely, is one of the fastest ways to lose patients. Being "agile" and "nimble" are more than just buzzwords bandied about by management consultants.

7. *Failure to set reasonable goals and timelines*: without a realistic working framework for its implementation, even the best strategic plan is pretty well useless. Strategic plans are a collection of action plans, each one of which consists of three key elements: a goal that will enhance the mission, action steps to reach the goal, and a timeline for achieving the goal that includes milestones. To ensure completion it also needs metrics to measure its achievement and someone who is responsible for monitoring them.

8. *Failure to put the plan into action*: the purpose of a strategic planning exercise is not just to create an impressive looking document with "Strategic Plan" written on its cover! No matter how many bullet point lists and coloured charts it includes, it cannot achieve spontaneous reality. Unless everyone tasked with its implementation buckles down and gets on with the job then it will all have been a waste of time.

9. *Lack of accountability*: there's a glaringly simple paradigm here; if no-one is held accountable then nothing will get done. Once the plan has been put into action there must be follow-up and follow-through. Specific individuals must be assigned areas of

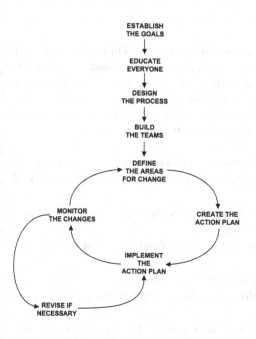

Figure 14.3 A road map of the journey to achieving excellence in the IVF lab.

accountability, allowed the authority and resources to achieve their goal(s), and made responsible for their particular area – but the plan needs to be shared openly with the entire team, and that way everyone can be held openly accountable. Most action plan elements fail due to inertia or passive resistance: achieving shared vision, buy-in and commitment are the keys to preventing these failures, but staff must be led, not ordered, to achieve change.

10. *Failure to monitor and follow-through*: if the plan for completing the actions contained in a strategic plan is just to have the clinic manager (or whoever has been made responsible by the clinic owner(s) or board of directors for its implementation) wait until everything has been reported to them as having been completed then it will be a very long wait! Progress with action items must be reviewed at regular – but not too frequent – intervals (e.g. quarterly, remember that a strategic plan is, by its nature, a long-term project, it won't be finished in just a few months!). These reviews must be formal, with agendas and minutes, and the minutes need to document not just progress but also next-step or revised action items and timelines. There is also a parallel truism for strategic plans that can be drawn from human conflict: "No campaign plan survives first contact with the enemy."

We have performed "operational performance reviews" of many ART labs around the world. Our reports have often included well over a hundred technical and operational recommendations (stratified as "must," "should," and "could" items), and when asked for advice on developing action plans we always start with the simple dictum "Don't bite off more than you can chew." Pick a few items that will give a good bang-for-the-buck, this will help everyone understand the value of change. Also select items with different timelines: don't just select several with expected big benefits that will all take a year to realize – include some (perhaps with more modest expected benefit) that can be completed sooner: then the value of the changes will start to become apparent sooner.

Is it all worth it?

Both of us have been intimately involved in accreditation systems and in taking private IVF centers through the accreditation process. We can, therefore, put our hands on our hearts and say, without reservation, that "Yes, it *is* all worth it." Yes, it does take a lot of time and effort, but these investments will be returned many-fold in the future as the lab, and the whole clinic, continues to operate "in control" and with the occurrence of crises greatly reduced. A true cost–benefit analysis will reveal that "quality always pays for itself" – in the long run.

As with everything in life, there is no guarantee of success or reward, but the benefits of embarking on the "quality journey" are irrefutable. There are also several highly beneficial corollaries to having a well-run IVF clinic.

- Keeping stress levels down for yourself and your staff by virtue of well-designed and efficient systems that are unlikely to go wrong.
- Being able to sleep easy at night, without having to worry about what went wrong today, or what might go wrong tomorrow.
- That warm glow that comes from "being the best."
- The comfort of knowing that you are unlikely to suffer the embarrassing catastrophes that befall some other clinics.
- The confidence that next time you're asked "What's wrong?" you'll be able to give the prompt response "Nothing, everything is running within its control limits." This is not about "CYA," but it certainly does give you asbestos underpants!

Implementing quality management and risk management in IVF centers should be based on carrots, and not sticks, but regulatory authorities will always have the last word: the EU Tissues and Cell Directive requires a formal quality management system, and so every IVF center in the EU has had to create one.

The extent to which quality management has been embraced within the global IVF community over the past decade is readily apparent. The European Society of Human Reproduction and Embryology (ESHRE) now not only has a Task Force on the EUTCD but also a Special Interest Group for Safety and Quality in ART. The American Society of Reproductive Medicine recently published in *Fertility and Sterility* a series of "Views and Reviews" articles on key topics in this area (Alper, 2013; de los Santos and Ruiz, 2013; de Ziegler *et al*, 2013; Meldrum and de Ziegler, 2013; Scott and De Ziegler, 2013). And the journal *Reproductive Biomedicine Online* has also initiated an ongoing Symposium on Quality Management in Assisted Reproductive Technology (Mortimer *et al.*, 2014; Swain, 2014).

Hopefully we have convinced you that professional self-respect should be sufficient motivation, and that prophylaxis is far better than cure.

References

Aitken RJ, Clarkson JS (1988) Significance of reactive oxygen species and antioxidants in defining the efficacy of sperm preparation techniques. *Journal of Andrology*, 9: 367–376.

Almeida PA, Bolton VN (1995) The effect of temperature fluctuations on the cytoskeletal organisation and chromosomal constitution of the human oocyte. *Zygote*, 3: 357–365.

Alper MM (2013) Experience with ISO quality control in assisted reproductive technology. *Fertility and Sterility* 100:1503–1508.

Alper MM, Brinsden PR, Fischer R, Wikland M (2002) Is your IVF programme good? *Human Reproduction*, 17: 8–10.

Alpha Scientists in Reproductive Medicine and ESHRE Special Interest Group of Embryology (2011a) The Istanbul consensus workshop on embryo assessment: proceedings of an expert meeting. *Reproductive Biomedicine Online* 22: 632–646 (simultaneous publication).

Alpha Scientists in Reproductive Medicine and ESHRE Special Interest Group of Embryology (2011b) The Istanbul consensus workshop on embryo assessment: proceedings of an expert meeting. *Human Reproduction* 26:1270–1283 (simultaneous publication).

Alpha Scientists in Reproductive Medicine (2012) The Alpha consensus meeting on cryopreservation key performance indicators (KPIs) and benchmarks: proceedings of an expert meeting directed by Alpha. *Reproductive Biomedicine Online* 25:146–167.

Asuero AM, Queraltó JM, Pujol-Ribera E *et al.* (2014) Effectiveness of a mindfulness education program in primary health care professionals: a pragmatic controlled trial. *Journal of Continuing Education in the Health Professions*, 34: 4–12.

Barratt CL, Björndahl L, Menkveld R, Mortimer D (2011) ESHRE special interest group for andrology basic semen analysis course: a continued focus on accuracy, quality, efficiency and clinical relevance. *Human Reproduction*, 26: 3207–3212.

Bavister BD (1995) Culture of preimplantation embryos: facts and artifacts. *Human Reproduction Update*, 1: 91–148.

Bavister BD (1999) Stage-specific culture media and reactions of embryos to them. In: Jansen R, Mortimer D (eds), *Towards Reproductive Certainty: Fertility and Genetics Beyond 1999*. Parthenon Publishing, Carnforth, Lancashire, UK, pp. 367–377.

Benson JD, Chicone CC, Critser JK (2012) Analytical optimal controls for the state constrained addition and removal of cryoprotective agents. *Bulletin of Mathematical Biology*, 74: 1516–1530.

Björndahl L (2011) What is normal semen quality? On the use and abuse of reference limits for the interpretation of semen analysis results. *Human Fertility*, 14: 179–186.

Björndahl L, Barratt CLR, Fraser LR, Kvist U, Mortimer D (2002) ESHRE basic semen analysis courses 1995–1999: immediate beneficial effects of standardized training. *Human Reproduction*, 17: 1299–1305.

Björndahl L, Mortimer D, Barratt CLR, *et al.* (2010) *A Practical Guide to Basic Laboratory Andrology*. Cambridge University Press, Cambridge.

Blake DA, Forsberg AS, Hillensjö T, Wikland M (1999) The practicalities of sequential blastocyst culture. Presented at *ART, Science and Fiction*, the Second International Alpha Congress, Copenhagen (Denmark), September 1999. debbie. blake@aut.ac.nz

Bogner MS (ed.) (1994) *Human Error In Medicine*. Lawrence Erlbaum Associates Inc, Hillsdale, NJ, USA.

Brison DR, Hooper M, Critchlow JD *et al.* (2004) Reducing risk in the IVF laboratory: implementation of a double witnessing system. *AVMA Medical and Legal Journal*, 10: 176–180.

Calman KC (1996) Cancer: science and society and the communication of risk. *British Medical Journal*, 313: 799–802.

Calman KC, Royston GHD (1997) Personal paper: risk language and dialects. *British Medical Journal*, 315: 939–942.

Canadian Standards Association (2012) *Z900.2.1–12: Tissues for Assisted Reproduction*. Ottawa, Canada.

Catt JW, Henman M (2000) Toxic effects of oxygen on human embryo development. *Human Reproduction*, 15, Suppl.2: 199–206.

Chian R-C, Quinn P (2010) *Fertility Cryopreservation*. Cambridge University Press, Cambridge, UK.

Cohen J (2013) On patenting time and other natural phenomena. *Reproductive Biomedicine Online*, 26: 109–110.

Cohen J, Gilligan A, Esposito W, Schimmel T, Dale B (1997) Ambient air and its potential effects on conception *in vitro*. *Human Reproduction*, 12: 1742–1749.

Cohen J, Medley G (2005) *Stop Working and Start Thinking: A Guide to Becoming a Scientist, second edition*. Taylor & Francis, Abingdon, UK, 150pp.

Cook RR (1999) *Assessment of Uncertainties in Measurement for Calibration and Testing Laboratories*. National Association of Testing Authorities, Sydney, Australia. 57pp.

Cook IVF (1999) *Cook Culture Systems: Instructions for Use*. Cook IVF, Eight Mile Plains, Qld, Australia.

Cooke S, Tyler JP, Driscoll G (2002) Objective assessments of temperature maintenance using *in vitro* culture techniques. *Journal of Assisted Reproduction and Genetics*,19: 368–375.

Coombs A (2001) *The Living Workplace: Soul, Spirit and Success in the 21st Century*. HarperCollins Publishers Ltd, Toronto, Canada, 188pp.

Cooper TG, Noonan E, von Eckardstein S *et al.* (2010) World Health Organization reference values for human semen characteristics. *Human Reproduction Update*, 16: 231–245.

Cullinan RT, Catt JW, Fussell S, Henman M, Mortimer D (1998) Improved implantation rates of cryopreserved human embryos thawed in a phosphate-free medium. 14th Annual Meeting of the European Society of Human Reproduction and Embryology, Göteborg (Sweden), June 1998. Abstract O-117. *Human Reproduction*, 13 (Abstract Book 1): 59–60.

Dale B, McQuater R (1998) *Managing Business Improvement and Quality: Implementing Key Tools and Techniques*. Blackwell Publishers, Oxford, UK.

Damelio R (1996) *The Basics of Process Mapping*. Productivity Inc, Portland, OR, USA.

de los Santos MZJ, Ruiz A (2013) Protocols for tracking and witnessing samples and patients in assisted reproductive technology. *Fertility and Sterility* 100:1499–1502.

DeMarco T (2001) *Slack: Getting Past Burnout, Busywork, and the Myth of Total Efficiency*. Broadway Books, New York, NY, USA.

Deming WE. *Out of the Crisis*. MIT, Cambridge, MA, USA, 1982, 1986.

de Ziegler D, Gambone JC, Meldrum DR, Chapron C (2013) Risk and safety management in infertility and assisted reproductive technology (ART): from the doctor's office to the ART procedure. *Fertility and Sterility*, 100:1509–1517.

Edwards R, Steptoe P (1980) *A Matter of Life*. Hutchinson & Co, London, UK.

Elder K, Elliott T (1998) *Problem Solving and Troubleshooting in IVF*. Ladybrook Publishing, Perth, WA, Australia.

Ford WCL, Rees JM (1990) The bioenergetics of mammalian sperm motility. In: Gagnon C (ed), *Controls of Sperm Motility: Biological and Clinical Aspects*. CRC Press, Boca Raton, FL, USA, pp. 175–202.

Fraser LR, Quinn PJ (1981) A glycolytic product is obligatory for initiation of the sperm acrosome reaction and whiplash motility required for fertilization in the mouse. *Journal of Reproduction and Fertility*, 61: 25–35.

George ML, Rowlands D, Proce M, Maxey J (2005) *The Lean Six Sigma Pocket Toolbook*. Mcraw-Hill, New York, NY, USA.

Gonen Y, Dirnfeld M, Goldman S, Koifman M, Abramovici H (1991) Does the choice of catheter for embryo transfer influence the success rate of *in-vitro* fertilization? *Human Reproduction*, 6:1092–1094.

Graban M, Swartz JE (2014) *The Executive Guide to Healthcare Kaizen: Leadership for a Continuously Learning and Improving Organization*. CRC Press, Boca Raton, FL, USA.

Grout JR (2004) Process mapping. URL: http://campbell.berry.edu/faculty/jgrout/processmapping/

Harbottle S (2003) Are You Working Too Hard? Annual Meeting of the Association of Clinical Embryologists, Glasgow (UK).

Heller R, Hindle T (2003) *Essential Manager's Manual*. DK Publishing, New York, NY, USA.

Hobbs P (2009) *Project Management*. DK Publishing, New York, NY, USA.

Hutchison D (1994) *Total Quality Management in the Clinical Laboratory*. ASQC Quality Press, Milwaukee, WI, USA.

IEEE Standards Association (1998) *IEEE Standard for Function Modeling Language – Syntax and Semantics for IDEF0. IEEE 1320.1-1998 (Replaces FIPS PUB 183)*. Institute of Electrical and Electronics Engineers Standards Association, Piscataway, NJ, USA. URL: http://standards.ieee.org/.

ISO (1993) *ISO/TS 14253-2:1999 Geometrical Product Specifications (GPS) – Inspection by measurement of workpieces and measuring equipment – Part 2: Guide to the estimation of uncertainty in GPS measurement, in calibration of measuring equipment and in product verification*. International Organization for Standardization, Geneva, Switzerland.

ISO (2008) *International standard ISO 9001:2008. Quality Management Systems – Requirements*. International Organization for Standardization, Geneva, Switzerland.

ISO (2011) *International Standard ISO 19011:2011. Guidelines for Auditing Management Systems*. International Organization for Standardization, Geneva, Switzerland.

ISO (2012) *International Standard ISO 15189:2012. Medical Laboratories – Requirements for quality and competence*. International Organization for Standardization, Geneva, Switzerland.

Jacka JM, Keller P (2001) *Business Process Mapping: Improving Customer Satisfaction*. John Wiley & Sons, Ltd, New York, NY, USA.

Kaser DJ, Racowsky C (2014) Clinical outcomes following selection of human preimplantation embryos with time-lapse monitoring: a systematic review. *Human Reproduction Update*, 20: 617-631.

Kennedy CR (2004) Risk management in assisted reproduction. *AVMA Medical and Legal Journal*, 10: 169-175.

Krafcik, JF (1988) Triumph of the lean production system. *Sloan Management Review* 30: 41-52.

Lane M, Lyons, MA, Bavister BD (2000) Cryopreservation reduces the ability of hamster 2-cell embryos to regulate intracellular pH. *Human Reproduction*, 15: 389-394.

Leape LL (1997) A systems analysis approach to medical error. *Journal of Evaluation in Clinical Practice*, 3: 213-222.

Leese HJ (1990) The environment of the preimplantation embryo. In: Edwards RG (ed), *Establishing a Successful Human Pregnancy*, Serono Symposia Publications Volume 66, Raven Press, New York, NY, USA, pp. 143-154.

Marconi G, Vilela M, Bello J, Diradourian M, Quintana R, Sueldo C (2003) Endometrial lesions caused by catheters used for embryo transfers: a preliminary report. *Fertility and Sterility*, 80: 363-367.

Mayer JF, Jones EL, Dowling-Lacey D *et al.* (2003) Total quality improvement in the IVF laboratory: choosing indicators of quality. *Reproductive Biomedicine Online*, 7: 695-699.

Mayer JF, Nehchiri F, Weedon VM *et al.* (1999) Prospective randomized crossover analysis of the impact of an IVF incubator air filtration system (Coda, GenX) on clinical pregnancy rates. *Fertility and Sterility*, Suppl.1: S42-S43.

McDonald JA, Norman RJ (2002) A randomized controlled trial of a soft double lumen embryo transfer catheter versus a firm single lumen catheter: significant improvements in pregnancy rates. *Human Reproduction*, 17:1502-1506.

Meldrum DR, de Ziegler D (2013) Introduction: Risk and safety management in infertility and assisted reproductive technology. *Fertility and Sterility*, 100 :1497-1498.

Menezo Y (1976) Milieu synthétique pour la survie et la maturation des gamètes et pour la culture de l'oeuf fécondé. *Comptes Rendus de l'Academie des Sciences de Paris, Série D*, 282:1967-1970.

Meriano J, Weissman A, Greenblatt EM, Ward S, Casper RF (2000) The choice of embryo transfer catheter affects embryo implantation after IVF. *Fertility and Sterility*, 74:678-682.

Meseguer M, Rubio I, Cruz M *et al.* (2012) Embryo incubation and selection in a time-lapse monitoring system improves pregnancy outcome compared with a standard incubator: a retrospective cohort study. *Fertility and Sterility*, 98: 1481–1489, e10.

Mortimer D (1986) Elaboration of a new culture medium for physiological studies on human sperm motility and capacitation. *Human Reproduction*, 1: 247–250.

Mortimer D (1991) Sperm preparation techniques and iatrogenic failures of in-vitro fertilization. *Human Reproduction*, 6: 173–176.

Mortimer D (1994) *Practical Laboratory Andrology*. Oxford University Press, New Tork, NY, USA, 393pp.

Mortimer D (1999) Quality management in the IVF laboratory. In: Jansen R, Mortimer D (eds), *Towards Reproductive Certainty: Fertility and Genetics Beyond 1999*. Parthenon Publishing, Carnforth, UK, pp. 421–426.

Mortimer D (2000) Sperm preparation methods. *Journal of Andrology*, 21: 357–366.

Mortimer D (2004a) Current and future concepts and practices in human sperm cryobanking. *Reproductive Biomedicine Online*, 9: 134–151.

Mortimer D (2004b) Setting up risk management systems in IVF laboratories. *Clinical Risk*, 10: 128–137.

Mortimer ST (2002) Practical application of computer-aided sperm analysis (CASA). In: van der Horst G, Franken D, Bornman R, de Jager T, Dyer S (eds), *Proceedings of the 9th International Symposium on Spermatology*, (Cape Town, South Africa). Monduzzi Editore S.p.A., Bologna, Italy, pp.233–238.

Mortimer, D, Barratt CLR (2006) Is there a real risk of transmitting variant Creutzfeldt-Jakob disease by donor sperm insemination? *Reproductive Biomedicine Online*, 13: 778–790.

Mortimer D, Demetriou A, Cullinan R, Henman M, Jansen RPS (1995) A novel approach to IVF laboratory quality control. IXth World Congress on In Vitro Fertilization and Assisted Reproduction, Vienna (Austria), April 1995, Abstract OC-160. *Journal of Assisted Reproduction and Genetics*, 12(3) Suppl: 66S.

Mortimer D, Di Berardino T (2008) To alarm or monitor? A cost-benefit analysis comparing laboratory dial-out alarms and a real-time monitoring system. *Alpha Newsletter*, No 39 (7 pages).

Mortimer D, Henman MJ, Jansen RPS (2002a) *Development of an Improved Embryo Culture System for Clinical Human IVF*. William A. Cook Australia, Eight Mile Plains, Qld, Australia.

Mortimer D, Mortimer ST (1992) Methods of sperm preparation for assisted reproduction. *Annals of the Academy of Medicine of Singapore*, 21: 517–524.

Mortimer D, Poole T, Cohen J (2014) Introduction to Quality Management in Assisted Reproductive Technology Symposium. *Reproductive Biomedicine Online*, 28:533–534.

Mortimer D, Shu MA, Tan R (1986) Standardization and quality control of sperm concentration and sperm motility counts in semen analysis. *Human Reproduction*, 1: 299–303.

Mortimer D, Shu MA, Tan R, Mortimer ST (1989) A technical note on diluting semen for the haemocytometric determination of sperm concentration. *Human Reproduction*, 4: 166–168.

Mortimer S, Fluker M, Yuzpe A (2001a) Keeping the lab in control: use of laboratory performance measures. 47th Annual Meeting of the Canadian Fertility and Andrology Society, Whistler (BC, Canada), Abstract FP3.

Mortimer S, Fluker M, Yuzpe A (2001b) Effect of culture conditions on embryo cleavage rates and morphology. 47th Annual Meeting of the Canadian Fertility and Andrology Society, Whistler (BC, Canada), Abstract FP1.

Mortimer, ST, Fluker MR, Yuzpe AA (2002b) Relative effects of culture conditions on fertilization rate and embryo quality. 48th Annual Meeting of the Canadian Fertility and Andrology Society, Manoir Richelieu (Quebec, Canada), Abstract FP23.

Mortimer, ST, Fluker MR, Yuzpe AA (2002c) Effect of embryo transfer catheter on implantation rates. *Fertility and Sterility*, 76(3S):S17–S18, Abstract O-045.

Munné S, Magli C, Adler A et al. (1997) Treatment-related chromosome abnormalities in human embryos. *Human Reproduction*, 12: 780–784.

Murray CT, Mortimer D (1999) Monitoring laboratory performance measures for quality assurance in IVF. 11th World Congress on In Vitro Fertilization and Human Reproductive Genetics, Sydney, Australia. Abstract O-058, p90.

National Institute of Standards and Technology (1993) Integration definition for function modelling (IDEF-0). Draft Federal Information Processing Standards Publication 183. Available from URL: http://www.idef.com/.

NCCLS (2002) Clinical Laboratory Technical Procedure Manuals; Approved Guideline – Fourth Edition, document GP2-A4. NCCLS, Wayne, PA, USA. URL: www.nccls.org

Pickering SJ, Braude PR, Johnson MH, Cant A, Currie J (1990) Transient cooling to room temperature can cause irreversible disruption of the meiotic spindle in the human oocyte. *Fertility and Sterility*, 54: 102–108.

Porath C, Pearson C (2009) How toxic colleagues corrode performance. *Harvard Business Review*, April: 24.

Quinn P (1995) Enhanced results in mouse and human embryo culture using a modified human tubal fluid medium lacking glucose and phosphate ions. *Journal of Assisted Reproduction and Genetics*, 12: 97–105.

Quinn P (ed) (2014) *Culture Media, Solutions, and Systems in Human ART*. Cambridge University Press, Cambridge, UK.

Quinn P, Kerin JF, Warnes GM (1985) Improved pregnancy rate in human in vitro fertilization with the use of a medium based on the composition of human tubal fluid. *Fertility and Sterility*, 44:493–498.

Reason JT (1994) Foreword. In: Bogner MS (ed), *Human Error in Medicine*. Lawrence Erlbaum Associates Inc, Hillsdale, NJ, USA.

Regehr C, Glancy D, Pitts A, Leblanc VR (2014) Interventions to reduce the consequences of stress in physicians: a review and meta-analysis. *Journal of Nervous and Mental Disease*, 202:353–359.

Sánchez-Pozo MC, Mendiola J, Serrano M et al.; Special Interest Group in Andrology of the European Society of Human Reproduction and Embryology (2013) Proposal of guidelines for the appraisal of SEMen QUAlity studies (SEMQUA). *Human Reproduction*, 28: 10–21.

Scott RT, De Ziegler N (2013) Could safety boards provide a valuable tool to enhance the safety of reproductive medicine? *Fertility and Sterility* 100:1518–1523.

Sharpe VA, Faden AI (1998) *Medical Harm: Historical, Conceptual, and Ethical Dimensions of Iatrogenic Illness*. Cambridge University Press, Cambridge, UK.

Shewhart WA (1986) *Statistical Method from the Viewpoint of Quality Control*. Dover Publications Inc, Mineola, NY, USA. (A reprint of the original edition published by the Graduate School of the Department of Agriculture, Washington, DC, 1939.)

Sinek S (2009) *Start with Why: How Great Leaders Inspire Everyone to Take Action*. Portfolio, a member of the Penguin Group (USA) Inc., NY, USA.

Sinek S (2014) *Leaders Eat Last: Why Some Teams Pull Together and Others Don't*. Penguin Group (USA) LLC, NY, USA.

Singleton O, Hölzel BK, Vangel M et al. (2014) Change in brainstem grey matter concentration following a mindfulness-based intervention is correlated with improvement in psychological well-being. *Frontiers in Human Neuroscience*, 8: 33.

Slovic P, Finucane ML, Peters E, MacGregor DG (2004) Risk as analysis and risk as feelings: some thoughts about affect, reason, risk, and rationality. *Risk Analysis*, 24, 311–322.

Stoop D, De Munck N, Jansen E et al. (2012) Clinical validation of a closed vitrification system in an oocyte-donation programme. *Reproductive Biomedicine Online*, 24: 180–185.

Swain J (2014) Decisions for the IVF laboratory: comparative analysis of embryo culture incubators. *Reproductive Biomedicine Online* 28:535–547.

Tedder RS, Zuckerman MA, Goldstone AH et al. (1995) Hepatitis B transmission from contaminated cryopreservation tank. *Lancet* 346, 137–140.

Tervit HR, Whittingham DG, Rowson LEA (1972) Successful culture in vitro of sheep and cattle ova. *Journal of Reproduction and Fertility*, 30: 493–497.

Testart J, Lassalle B, Frydman R (1982) Apparatus for the in vitro fertilization and culture of human oocytes. *Fertility and Sterility*, 38: 372–375.

Thornhill AR, Orriols Brunetti X, Bird S (2013) Measuring human error in the IVF laboratory using an electronic witnessing system. *Proceedings of the 17th World Congress on Controversies in Obstetrics, Gynecology and Infertility, Lisbon, Portugal, 2013.* Monduzzi Editoriali, Bologna, pp101–106.

Toft B, Mascie-Taylor H (2005) Involuntary automaticity: a work-system induced risk to sage health care. *Health Services Management Research*, 18: 211–216.

Van Landuyt L, Stoop D, Verheyen G *et al.* (2011) Outcome of closed blastocyst vitrification in relation to blastocyst quality: evaluation of 759 warming cycles in a single-embryo transfer policy. *Human Reproduction*, 26: 527–534.

van Weering, HGI, Schats R, McDonnell J *et al.* (2002) The impact of the embryo transfer catheter on the pregnancy rate in IVF. *Human Reproduction,*17:666–670.

Wang WH, Meng L, Hackett RJ, Odenbourg R, Keefe DL (2001) Limited recovery of meiotic spindles in living human oocytes after cooling-rewarming observed using polarized light microscopy. *Human Reproduction*, 16: 2374–2378.

Wikland M, Sjoblom C (2000) The application of quality systems in ART programs. *Molecular and Cellular Endocrinology*, 166: 3–7.

Wilson K. 10 Ways to Kill Your Strategic Plan. See http://blog.smartdraw.com/10-ways-kill-strategic-plan/ (accessed 06/02/2014).

Wisanto A, Camus M, Janssens R *et al.* (1989) Performance of different embryo transfer catheters in a human in vitro fertilization program. *Fertility and Sterility*, 52:79–84.

World Health Organization (1999) *WHO Laboratory Manual for the Examination of Human Semen and Sperm-Cervical Mucus Interaction, fourth edition.* Cambridge University Press, Cambridge, UK.

World Health Organization (2010) *WHO Laboratory Manual for the Examination and Processing of Human Semen, fifth edition.* Cambridge University Press, Cambridge, UK.

Index

Printed in the United States
By Bookmasters